Reducing READMISSIONS

A Blueprint for Improving Care Transitions

Christina Pavetto Bond, MS, FACHE

Eric A. Coleman, MD, MPH

HCPro

Reducing Readmissions: A Blueprint for Improving Care Transitions is published by HCPro, Inc.

Christina Pavetto Bond, MS, FACHE, Author
Eric A. Coleman, MD, MPH, Author
Janet Morris, Senior Managing Editor
Ilene MacDonald, Executive Editor
Lauren McLeod, Group Publisher

Mike Mirabello, Senior Graphic Artist
Amanda Lautieri, Proofreader
Matt Sharpe, Production Supervisor
Susan Darbyshire, Art Director
Jean St. Pierre, Senior Director of Operations

Advice given is general. Readers should consult professional counsel for specific legal, ethical, or clinical questions. Arrangements can be made for quantity discounts. For more information, contact:

HCPro, Inc.
P.O. Box 1168
Marblehead, MA 01945
Telephone: 800/650-6787 or 781/639-1872
Fax: 800/639-8511
E-mail: *customerservice@hcpro.com*

Visit HCPro online at:
www.hcpro.com and www.hcmarketplace.com

Contents

About the Authors

Christina Pavetto Bond, MS, FACHE

Christy Bond, MS, FACHE, is the founding director of a service line focused on aging and complex care at Crouse Hospital in Syracuse, NY. In this role, she has introduced several best-practice programs, including NICHE (Nurses Improving the Care of Healthsystem Elders), HELP (Hospital Elder Life Program), the Care Transitions Intervention^SM, and the Transitional Care Model. In addition, Christy has led her hospital's participation in several grant-funded national collaboratives, including the Medicare Innovations Collaborative, to develop strategies for integrating best-practice geriatric care, and Stop CAUTI, to reduce catheter-associated urinary tract infections. She has also led her hospital's participation in four regional collaboratives to improve care transitions focused on community-dwelling elders, patients in long-term care, and adults with sensory loss and caregivers.

Christy also has experience at an academic medical system. As the quality administrator, she led the development and implementation of the organization's strategic quality plan and managed departments charged with supporting quality efforts, including clinical practice analysis, infection control, risk management, case management, and guest services.

A fellow in the American College of Healthcare Executives and a board-certified hospital administrator, Christy has extensive experience in clinical program development, role design, quality improvement leadership, and educational programming. With degrees in business administration and education, she is a frequently invited speaker on the business development of a geriatric service line, leadership, and patient self-management.

Christy lives in Central New York with her sons, Stephen and Jonathan.

Eric A. Coleman, MD, MPH

Eric A. Coleman, MD, MPH, is professor of medicine within the Divisions of Health Care Policy and Research and Geriatric Medicine at the University of Colorado at Denver and Health Sciences Center. Dr. Coleman is the director of the Care Transitions Program^{SM}, aimed at improving quality and safety during times of care "handoffs." He is also the executive director of the Practice Change Fellows Program, designed to build leadership capacity among healthcare professionals who are responsible for geriatric programs and service lines.

Dr. Coleman bridges innovation and practice through: (1) enhancing the role of patients and caregivers in improving the quality of their care transitions across acute and postacute settings; (2) measuring quality of care transitions from the perspective of patients and caregivers; (3) implementing system-level practice improvement interventions; and (4) using health information technology to promote safe and effective care transitions.

For more information, please go to *www.caretransitions.org* or *www.practicechangefellows.org.*

Acknowledgments

The first person whose contribution I must acknowledge is Dr. Eric Coleman. Dr. Coleman taught me it is imperative for hospitals to ensure patients are safely received at the next level of care. And the secret is to empower the patient. Thank you, Dr. Coleman, for your guidance. I am honored to begin this book with your chapter.

Programs developed by some of the most inspired minds and dedicated clinicians in healthcare are discussed in this book. I am honored to be able to write about their work. Thank you, Dr. Coleman, creator of the Care Transitions Intervention^{SM}, Dr. Mary Naylor, creator of the Transitional Care Program, and Dr. Brian Jack, creator of Project RED, for reviewing your chapters. Also, thank you to Brian Bixby for educating me about Dr. Naylor's program. And thanks to Lynn Schipelliti and Kimberly Visconti at Boston Medical for reviewing the chapter on Project RED and clarifying your process.

Dr. Judith Hibbard has developed what I think is an essential assessment for the patient education and coaching process. Thank you for reviewing the information on the Patient Activation Measure. Thank you, Chris Delaney, for facilitating Dr. Hibbard's participation.

I am fortunate to work with a team of nurses who have repeatedly joined me in the journey to implementing unique improvements in care. Thank you, Cindy, Sharon, and Diane for your enthusiasm and professionalism each day. And thank you for reviewing some of the case studies.

Thank you very much, Stephanie. Your creative genius made me a much better writer and led to the perfect name for this book. And Denise, the nurse I always turn to, thank you for reviewing some of the case studies.

Finally, I must thank my mentor, Mike Eesley, for teaching me about true leadership and trusting me to do it well.

Dedication

To my sons, Stephen and Jonathan, and my mother Shirley—you are my inspiration.

Introduction

In reading this book, you and I share a common interest in improving the health and well-being of the patients we serve. My background and, thus, my approach to this undertaking are unique. Approximately 20 years ago, I made the transition from teaching college students about business and leadership to healthcare administration. Whenever possible, I drew from my background in education to enhance what I was doing as a healthcare administrator. This book contains practical information that I found useful in implementing transitions programming to reduce readmissions. But you will also find information on the patient education process that may be different from what you are used to. I urge you to view it with an open mind and think about your experiences with patients when you read it. I am certain you will find that it enhances your perceptions about patients as adult learners in the discharge and transitions processes.

Because I am administrator now, my life is implementing new programs. So, I have included strategic discussions of the benefits of transitions programming and considerations for implementation. I have also tried to provide you with practical tools you can adapt and use right away as you begin to implement these programs. To enhance your experience, I have included tips from some of the greatest minds in business and leadership. They are not all healthcare leaders, but I think a broader base of knowledge helps us think more creatively about solutions to healthcare problems. I know the best ideas often originate with frontline staff and people in informal leadership roles. If you are in that position, I hope you find the case studies helpful in thinking about the practical aspects of functioning in a transitions role.

Inside this book you will find a wide-ranging, yet succinct, review of some of the strongest programming to reduce readmissions that exists today, as well as discussions of many corresponding issues. I hope you find it comprehensive enough to allow you to begin the process of adoption in your facility.

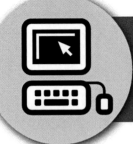

DOWNLOAD YOUR MATERIALS NOW

These customizable tools are available to download:

- Program Budget Sample

- Transition Program Outcome Tracking Tool

- A Checksheet for Implementation

- Discharge Advocate Sample Job Description

- Transition Coach Sample Job Description

You will find them at the URL below.

www.hcpro.com/downloads/8534

Thank you for purchasing this product!

HCPro

Time to Reinvent Transitional Care for Older Adults?

LEARNING OBJECTIVES

After reading this chapter, you should be able to:

- Identify the leading components of quality transitional care

- Explain the role healthcare technology should play in enhancing the transition process

by:

Eric A. Coleman, MD, MPH
Director, Care Transitions Program
Professor of Medicine
University of Colorado at Denver

The goal of this chapter is to provide a framework for reinventing transitional care that will set the stage for subsequent chapters, which will explore the transition approaches of a distinguished collection of leaders in the field. The chapter will conclude with an overview of promising directions in national health policy that may serve to better align incentives for delivering high-quality transitional care services.

Definition of Transitional Care

The term *transitional care* has evolved to include many connotations in healthcare delivery. For the purpose of this chapter, we will derive the definition of transitional care from the American Geriatrics Society:

"A set of actions designed to ensure the coordination and continuity of healthcare as patients transfer

between different locations or different levels of care within the same location. Representative locations include (but are not limited to) hospitals, sub-acute and post-acute nursing facilities, the patient's home, primary and specialty care offices, and long-term care facilities. Transitional care is based on a comprehensive plan of care and the availability of healthcare practitioners who are well trained in chronic care and have current information about the patient's goals, preferences, and clinical status. It includes logistical arrangements, education of the patient and family, and coordination among the health professionals involved in the transition. Transitional care, which encompasses both the sending and the receiving aspects of the transfer, is essential for persons with complex care needs."[1]

A Need for a Galvanizing Vision

Although transitional care is a critical component of quality care and safety for older adults, it suffers from the lack of a clear and galvanizing vision shared by consumers, family caregivers, health professionals, and policy makers.

Current challenges include controversy over which elements of transitional care coordination are most essential, wide variation in program design and execution, a prevailing provider-centric orientation, and conflicting evidence from existing trials as to whether transitional care improves outcomes and reduces costs. At a more fundamental level, do we conceptualize transitional care as a set of services? A detailed assessment and care plan? A particular healthcare professional that spans different care settings? Given the attention care coordination in general and transitional care in particular is receiving in policy discussions, now would seem to be a critical time to articulate a practice change vision.

Increasing evidence suggests widespread problems associated with the quality of transitional care. One in five Medicare beneficiaries is rehospitalized within 30 days, costing our nation more than $17 billion annually.[2] The lack of incentives and accountability make these transfers particularly susceptible to medical errors, service duplication, and unnecessary utilization.[3] Consumers are uniquely positioned to reflect upon the quality of transitional care, acknowledging that they are often the only common thread weaving across an episode of chronic illness exacerbation. Qualitative studies have consistently shown that patients and their caregivers do not know what to expect and are unprepared for their role in the next care setting. They do not understand essential steps in the management of their condition, feel abandoned because they do not know which healthcare practitioner to contact for guidance, and believe that their input into their care plan is often disregarded. Many patients and caregivers are frustrated with the significant amount of redundancy in assessments and dissatisfied with having to perform tasks that their healthcare practitioners have left undone.[4]

Optimal transitional care begins with consumer engagement as active participants in their care. This vision further encompasses a targeting approach designed to identify those individuals at high risk for poor quality transitional care, a measurement strategy to evaluate the effectiveness of interventions from the standpoint of payers, clinicians, and consumers, and employs interoperable health information technology to foster timely and accurate information exchange. Optimal transitional care requires an alignment of financial incentives and removal of regulatory impediments. Ultimately, transitional care can be characterized as providing the right care in the right place at the right time by consumers, family caregivers, and healthcare professionals with the right skill sets, and at a price that promotes the long-term sustainability of our healthcare financial resources.

Engage consumers

The value of engaging consumers—patients and family caregivers—as active participants in their transitional care has not received adequate national attention. Engagement includes coaching to promote skill transfer and activation to express treatment preferences and ensure that needs are met. Consumers live with their chronic conditions 24 hours per day, seven days per week. In most cases, their illness exacerbations and their attempts to respond to common transitional care challenges occur when no healthcare professionals are present. If this is not reason enough to engage consumers, consider the impending healthcare professional workforce shortage exacerbated by our aging population detailed in the recent Institute of Medicine (IOM) report. In 2010, the first cohort of baby boomers will reach the age of 65.[5] Thus, engaging consumers is not only the right thing to do, it has become a necessity.

However, we have a long road ahead to achieve this worthy aim of consumer engagement. As an illustration, the results of the Centers for Medicare & Medicaid Services (CMS) Medicare Care Coordination Demonstration were released in 2009.[6] Among the 15 individual trials conducted in exemplary health delivery systems, 14 did not show improved outcomes or reduced costs. None of the trials explicitly focused on consumer engagement of patients or family caregivers, and none focused on family caregiver training and involvement.

Fortunately, the United Hospital Fund's Next Step in Care *(www.nextstepincare.org)* provides family caregivers with guides to hospital discharge, medication management, and other navigation tools. Meanwhile, health coaching is gaining greater attention as an effective strategy to engage consumers as more active participants in their care, as well as to impart the skills and confidence they need to ensure they receive what they need. Health coaching has been used in a wide variety of programs and models with goals such as helping patients:

1. Manage a specific condition (such as diabetes);

2. Navigate a process (such as cancer treatment);

3. Be more informed and engaged in their healthcare (communication and information focus); and/or

4. Achieve specific health or wellness goals.[7-11]

A more expansive discussion of transitional care coaching follows in Chapter 5.

Targeting

Beginning with the rationale that most interventions designed to improve quality are time- and resource-intensive, our national health budget simply cannot afford to provide these to every patient undergoing transitions. Enter the need for a targeting strategy to identify those individuals who are at the highest risk to then tailor limited resources to those with the greatest need. Within the context of such decision-making, the nature and magnitude of the risk is often implied and therefore not readily apparent. Risk can be defined from different perspectives. For example, health insurers often equate risk in terms of likelihood for future use of high-cost healthcare services such as hospitalization. Alternatively, clinicians may conceptualize risk from the standpoint of likelihood for poor quality care or adverse medical events such as medication errors. From the consumer's perspective, risk could be envisioned as the likelihood of not receiving the necessary services for managing one's condition.

What is often lacking from each of these views of risks and many others is the extent to which this risk can be mitigated. In other words, can the trajectory of the downward spiral be modified with a well-placed intervention? For example, patients who are requiring high-intensity, high-cost services are unlikely to remain on this course for long—typically, either they improve or they die. Let's explore a number of approaches commonly undertaken to target high-risk patients for transition-related services.

The use of administrative data represents an attractive approach to risk identification. Health plans and governmental agencies often gravitate toward this strategy. Once collected, these data sets offer a wealth of valuable information on demographics, diagnoses, medication use, and prior healthcare utilization to construct risk indexes. Although many of these risk tools have been developed for routine use[12] (*www.acmq.org/natlconf/pdfs/goldfield.pdf*), this approach is constrained by a number of limitations. The first was alluded to earlier; these risk indexes do not tell us much about modifiable risk. A potential exception is the strategy to target based on admission for an ambulatory sensitive condition.[13] These are conditions for which it is hypothesized that earlier treatment-seeking behavior to a primary care source could have led to intervention to avert the hospital admission. The second is that there are patient characteristics that are of potential great importance to determining risk that are not routinely available in administrative databases, including presence of a willing and able family caregiver, financial or transportation barriers to obtaining one's medications, and whether the individual has a reliable source of primary care.

In 2009, CMS began publicly reporting hospitals' 30-day readmission rates for Medicare beneficiaries discharged for congestive heart failure, acute myocardial infarction, and pneumonia (*www.hospitalcompare. hhs.gov*). Given that hospitals now have greater incentive to improve their performance for these three conditions, it follows that this initiative may drive their approach to targeting.

Beyond using diagnostic criteria, targeting could also be directed toward those patients at greatest risk for poor comprehension or execution of their discharge instructions. With support from the Aetna Foundation, our Care Transitions Program℠ led an effort to guide healthcare leaders in this manner.[14] Developed through a comprehensive review of the literature, individual conversations with leaders in the field, and the convening of an expert panel, we articulated a multi-tiered prototypical approach that could be tailored to the resources of a given provider or health plan. Within the first tier, we recommend the use of the teach-back method and the clock-drawing test for detecting low health literacy and impaired cognitive function respectively. At the second level, we recommend the use of simulation of specific actions included in discharge instructions to allow more in-depth assessment as to whether the patient is likely to be able to carry out the discharge instructions.

The Society of Hospital Medicine provides leadership for project BOOST (Better Outcomes for Older adults through Safe Transitions) *(www.hospitalmedicine.org/boost)*. This project provides a framework for ensuring safe transitions for hospitalized Medicare beneficiaries, and its developers have proposed an approach to targeting based on the "7 Ps," which are:

- Problem medications

- Punk (i.e., depression)

- Principal diagnosis

- Polypharmacy

- Poor health literacy

- Patient support

- Prior hospitalization

The 7 Ps approach is based upon empirical research as well as clinical experience *(www.hospitalmedicine.org/ResourceRoomRedesign/RR_CareTransitions/CT_Home.cfm)*. Under ideal circumstances, the hospital care team is already assessing each of these items individually as part of the intake assessment. Aggregating across the seven factors then provides a more complete picture of a patient's overall risk.

Some healthcare organizations may choose to target based on the professional opinion of hospitalists, hospital nurses, discharge planners, or case managers to determine which patients are at high risk for poor quality care transitions. Although neither rigorous nor evidence-based, this type of approach may have a role in supplementing the other targeting approaches described.

The mentioned approaches attempt to identify risk but do not provide a clear path for how healthcare professionals may tailor information and services to reduce risk of subsequent preventable use of high-cost healthcare services. In contrast, the Patient Activation Measure (PAM) not only facilitates the ascertainment of risk, it further directs healthcare professionals on how to mitigate the risk.[15] The

PAM characterizes patient level of activation into four discrete categories. Once the category has been determined, the developers of the PAM provide guidance for how to measure both the amount and the approach for how to optimize the provision of patient instructions. The authors of the PAM have demonstrated that knowledge of patient activation combined with a directed intervention can both improve clinical indicators and reduce subsequent utilization.[16]

Measurement

The lack of quality measurement of transitional care represents a significant barrier to improving quality and safety. With few exceptions, quality is not routinely measured, and when it is, the focus is often on those elements of care provision that can be routinely ascertained and with minimal effort. Resistance often stems from the fact that no single healthcare setting "owns" transitional care, and therefore our setting-specific approach to quality measurement seems misapplied. The assignment of accountability often follows performance measurement and in the case of transitional care, this has heretofore been unclear. In 2009, a consensus statement on behalf of six leading physician professional societies released a set of standards that addressed this critical gap, articulating the nature and duration of accountability.[17] Although a detailed analysis of this topic is beyond the scope of this chapter, a comprehensive review can be found in a report from the IOM.[18] Since the release of the IOM report, a number of esteemed quality improvement efforts have revisited this important topic that will serve as the primary focus for this discussion.

3-Item Care Transitions Measure (CTM-3™)

The 3-Item Care Transitions Measure (CTM-3), developed by our Care Transitions Program[SM], was re-endorsed by the National Quality Forum for use in public reporting (*www.caretransitions.org/ctm_main.asp*). The measure has been translated into seven languages, and more than 3,000 organizations in 15 countries have requested permission for its use. Developed with direct input from consumers, the CTM-3 measures the extent to which patients are prepared for subsequent self-management of their health conditions. In this respect, the CTM-3 represents patient self-reported assessment of the quality of their care experience. This characteristic of the measure often attracts resistance on the part of healthcare providers who argue that patients are not able to judge the quality of their care experience. To counter these arguments, we have demonstrated that low CTM-3 scores strongly predict subsequent utilization.[19] Based on this finding, some of the CTM-3 adopters have employed this tool as a risk-screen at the time of hospital discharge.

HCAHPS

All hospitals are mandated by CMS to report their scores on the standardized Hospital Consumer Assessment of Health Plans (HCAHPS). Two of the HCAHPS survey items address hospital discharge. Like the CTM-3, HCAHPS is consumer-reported and has also been endorsed by the National Quality Forum. In contrast to the CTM-3 that measures the extent to which patients' sense of preparation for self-care, HCAHPS inquires as to whether patients recall receiving particular key information from their healthcare professionals:

- During your hospital stay, did hospital staff talk with you about whether you would have the help you needed when you left the hospital?

- During your hospital stay, did you get information in writing about what symptoms or health problems to look out for after you left the hospital?

The mandatory reporting program for 30-day hospital readmission enacted by CMS was described in the previous section on targeting. To date, this effort represents the ambitious attempt at wide-scale performance measurement reporting. Consumers who have the ability to select their preferred hospital can now make more informed decisions regarding which hospitals perform well on a range of factors, including the likelihood of readmission. Despite the fact that the reported measures have been risk-adjusted based largely on patient comorbidities, many hospitals and quality improvement experts believe there are many additional important factors that need to be taken into account, such as socio-economic status, race and ethnicity, and functional status.[20] These hospitals argue that failing to take these factors into account disadvantages those hospitals that disproportionately care for the nation's poor and underserved populations.

The American Medical Association (AMA) developed a series of recommended approaches for transitional care within the physician consortium performance improvement (PCPI) initiative. These approaches largely focus on recommended care processes that if done correctly would be hypothesized to result in improved quality of care. Most if not all of these approaches have not been formally evaluated for their measurement properties and may therefore be best characterized as a series of best practices. Because most practice settings continue to document these care approaches in paper medical records, determining how to collect information on these care processes remains a challenge (*www.ama-assn.org/ama/pub/physician-resources/clinical-practice-improvement/clinical-quality/physician-consortium-performance-improvement.shtml*).

Similarly, the American Medical Directors Association (AMDA) recently produced a comprehensive report on clinical practice guidelines for transitional care that are uniquely directed at the long-term care arena. As with the AMA PCPI approaches, the AMDA guidelines could be translated into processes of care that are relevant to the patients in nursing homes, long-term acute care hospitals, assisted living facilities, and adult day health programs.[21]

The National Transitions of Care Coalition (NTOCC) represents a diverse group of stakeholders, including healthcare professionals, national quality improvement entities, consumer groups, and insurers. NTOCC recently produced a practical step-by-step guide to help health organizations approach quality improvement (*www.ntocc.org/Portals/0/ImplementationPlan.pdf*).

Finally, although not explicitly designed to assess transitional care quality, the CMS Continuity Assessment and Record and Evaluation (CARE) tool provides an important infrastructure or platform from which quality can be measured (*www.pacdemo.rti.org*). The CARE tool would ultimately replace the site-specific assessment tools used in hospitals, nursing homes, and home care agencies in favor of a single assessment that would simply be validated and updated as patients move across care settings. The primary advantage of this tool is that for the first time, quality could potentially be evaluated across an entire episode of care.

The Role of Health Information Technology

Care fragmentation remains a significant threat to improving transitional care. The IOM report, *Crossing the Quality Chasm*, summarizes current practice, "Physician groups, hospitals and other healthcare organizations operate as silos, often providing care without the benefit of complete information about the patient's condition, medical history, services provided in other settings, or medications prescribed by other clinicians." In an ideal system, a core set of health information would seamlessly follow the patient between sites of care and include medications, allergies, a problem list, baseline function, advance directives, and family caregiver roles and contact information. The information would be updated across sites as test results become available, or as the healthcare needs of the patient change. The information would be secure, yet transparent to all involved in the care of the patient, whether it is the practitioner, patient, or caregiver. To date, however, we are far from realizing the potential that technology has to offer. To achieve this vision, financial incentives need to be in place to encourage health systems to adopt interoperable electronic health information systems, as hospitals and ambulatory clinics have been more likely to implement electronic medical records than nursing homes and home care agencies.[22]

In addition to interoperability, quality improvement in primary care will also be enhanced by mandatory e-prescribing and the implementation of unique patient identifiers. With regard to the former, wide-scale e-prescribing would facilitate the opportunity for each prescribing physician to see the complete list of medications a patient has received. With a more complete medication list, pharmacists would be better equipped to detect dangerous drug-drug interactions. Once all patients have an assigned unique patient identifier and healthcare utilization and testing information is collected into a single repository, health-care professionals can quickly determine which laboratory and diagnostic imaging tests have been recently performed and thereby avoid costly duplication.[23]

Aside from electronic medical records, two other health information facilitators include telehealth and the personal health record (PHR). Telehealth involves the use of technology to remotely engage and evaluate patients, particularly those who live in rural or frontier settings. The Veterans Affairs has been a leader in this regard (*www.carecoordination.va.gov/telehealth*). PHRs facilitate better cross-setting communication and encourage patients to own and routinely update a core set of health information. PeaceHealth's Shared Care Plan represents an important prototype (*www.sharedcareplan.org*). Microsoft Health Vault (*www.healthvault.com*) and Google Health (*www.google.com/health*) represent two of the nation's leaders in encouraging the use of PHRs by developing readily available, user-friendly platforms.

Finally, there is an important role for health information technology in what could be characterized as the ultimate in anticipatory transitional care: disaster preparation. Hurricane Katrina exposed the many weaknesses of our health information system.[24] Persons with multiple chronic conditions and nursing home residents were displaced without any record of their current problems, medications, or family caregivers.

The Policy Landscape

The statement "the only constant is change" embodies the current policy landscape regarding transitional care. Given the rapid state of flux, this section will focus on those areas that are likely to be central to policy efforts for the foreseeable future—namely controlling escalating healthcare costs, aligning financial incentives to improve quality, fostering greater accountability, and expanding the healthcare workforce. Fortunately, transitional care has garnered considerable national attention from leading quality improvement entities. These organizations include:

+ The Joint Commission

+ CMS and their quality improvement organizations

+ The Institute for Healthcare Improvement

+ The IOM

+ The National Quality Forum

+ The Medicare Payment Advisory Committee

+ The National Coalition on Care Coordination

The Obama administration and the U.S. Congress have clearly signaled intent to reign in escalating healthcare costs. Among potential targets for cost reduction, none is more attractive than the potential to reduce avoidable hospital readmissions. With an annual price tag estimated at $17 billion for the Medicare population, there is no other readily identified component of healthcare spending that could produce such a sizable return.[25] As previously stated, one in five Medicare beneficiaries is readmitted to the hospital within 30 days, representing an unequivocal failure to appropriately design and execute effective transitional care strategies. The Medicare Payment Advisory Commission that advises the Congress on changes to the Medicare program has proposed financial penalties for those hospitals with high readmission rates.[26]

Complementing strategies to drastically reduce healthcare spending are those approaches designed to align incentives for improving greater cross-setting coordination and collaboration, particularly for those patients transitioning across different care settings. In the past several years, three promising financing models were designed and are being piloted to better align these financial incentives, including the patient-centered medical home, bundled payment, and accountable care organizations. For a practice to be deemed a patient-centered medical home (and be eligible for additional payment), it must meet requirements developed by the National Committee for Quality Assurance (*www.ncqa.org/tabid/631/default.aspx*). These requirements include specific language for facilitating cross-setting care coordination. A second strategy involves providing hospitals and physician groups a single "bundled" payment to foster greater collaboration for managing recently discharged patients. CMS recently reported on a pilot study of this bundled payment approach.[27] Third, accountable care organizations extend the bundled payment concept across a community of healthcare providers and patients, thereby encouraging a more population-based approach to resource allocation to promote health inclusive of preventive treatment and restorative healthcare service delivery.

Summary

As the topic of transitional care increasingly becomes a central area of focus for both quality improvement and cost containment, your healthcare organization may benefit from the framework identified in this chapter to guide your decision-making. This chapter has provided such a framework for reinventing transitional care to serve this purpose, as well as to set the stage for subsequent chapters.

References

1. E.A. Coleman, C. Boult, American Geriatrics Society Health Care Systems Committee, "Improving the Quality of Transitional Care for Persons with Complex Care Needs," *Journal of the American Geriatrics Society*, 51 (2003): 556–57.

2. S.F. Jencks, M.V. Williams, E.A. Coleman, "Rehospitalization Among Patients in the Medicare Fee-for-Service Program," *The New England Journal of Medicine*, 360 (2009): 1418–28.

3. E.A. Coleman, R.A. Berenson, "Lost in Transition: Challenges and Opportunities for Improving the Quality of Transitional Care," *Annals of Internal Medicine*, 141 (2004): 533–36.

4. E.A. Coleman, E. Mahoney, C. Parry, "Assessing the Quality of Preparation for Posthospital Care from the Patient's Perspective: The Care Transitions Measure," *Medical Care*, 43 (2005): 246–55.

5. Institute of Medicine, *Retooling for an Aging America: Building the Healthcare Workforce*, (Washington, DC: The National Academies Press, 2008).

6. D. Peikes, A. Chen, J. Schore, R. Brown, "Effects of Care Coordination on Hospitalization, Quality of Care, and Health Care Expenditures Among Medicare Beneficiaries: 15 Randomized Trials," *The Journal of the American Medical Association*, 301 (2009): 603–18.

7. M.J. Vale, M. Jelinek, J. Best, A. Dart, L. Grigg, D. Hare, et al., "Coaching Patients On Achieving Cardiovascular Health (COACH): A Multicenter Randomized Trial in Patients with Coronary Heart Disease," *Archives of Internal Medicine*, 163 (2003): 2775–83.

8. R. Whittemore, G. Melkus, A. Sullivan, M. Grey, "A Nurse-Coaching Intervention for Women with Type 2 Diabetes," *The Diabetes Educator*, 30 (2004): 795–804.

9. G. Foster, S. Taylor, S. Eldridge, J. Ramsay, C. Griffiths, "Self-Management Education Programmes by Lay Leaders for People with Chronic Conditions," *Cochrane Database of Systematic Reviews*, Issue 4. Art. No. (2007): CD005108. DOI: 10.1002/14651858.CD005108.pub2.

10. A.M. Adelman, M. Graybill, "Integrating a Health Coach into Primary Care: Reflections from the Penn State Ambulatory Research Network," *Annals of Family Medicine*, 3 (2005): S33–S35.

11. M. Huffman M, "Health Coaching: A New and Exciting Technique to Enhance Patient Self-Management and Improve Outcomes," *Home Healthcare Nurse*, 25 (2007): 271-74.

12. D.G. Mosley, E. Peterson, D.C. Martin, "Do Hierarchical Condition Catergory Model Scores Predict Hospitalization Risk in Newly Enrolled Medicare Advantage Participants as Well as Probability of Repeated Admission Scores?" *Journal of American Geriatrics Society*, 57 (2009): 2306–10.

13. A.S. Bierman et al., "Ambulatory Care Sensitive Conditions: Ready for Prime Time?" Abstract. *Journal of General Internal Medicine*, 14 (1999): 88.

14. A. Chugh, M.V. Williams, J. Grigsby, E. Coleman, "Better Transitions: Improving Comprehension of Discharge Instructions," *Frontiers of Health Services Management*, 25 (2009): 11–32.

15. J.H. Hibbard, J. Stockard, E. Mahoney, M. Tusler, "Development of the Patient Activation Measure (PAM): Conceptualizing and Measuring Activation in Patients and Consumers," *Health Services Research*, 39 (2004): 1005–26.

16. J.H. Hibbard, J. Greene, M. Tusler, "Improving the Outcomes of Disease Management by Tailoring Care to the Patient's Level of Activation," *The American Journal of Managed Care*, 15 (2009):353–60.

17. V. Snow, D. Beck, T. Budnitz, D. Miller, J. Potter, R. Wears, et al., "Transitions of Care Consensus Policy Statement: American College of Physicians, Society of General Internal Medicine, Society of Hospital Medicine, American Geriatrics Society, American College of Emergency Physicians, and Society of Academic Emergency Medicine," *Journal of Hospital Medicine*, 4 (2009): 364–70.

18. E.A. Coleman, "Transitional Care Performance Measurement," *Commissioned Paper in Performance Measurement: Accelerating Improvement*, Committee on Redesigning Health Insurance Performance Measures, Payment, and Performance Improvement Programs, Institute of Medicine (Washington, DC: The National Academies Press, 2006), 250–86.

19. E.A. Coleman, C. Parry, S. Chalmers, A. Chugh, E. Mahoney, "The Central Role of Performance Measurement in Improving the Quality of Transitional Care," *Home Health Care Services Quarterly*, 26 (2007): 93–104.

20. R. Bhalla, G. Kalkut, "Could Medicare Readmission Policy Exacerbate Healthcare System Inequity?" *Annals of Internal Medicine*, 152 (2010): 114–17.

21. American Medical Directors Association, Transitions of Care in the Long-Term Care Continuum Clinical Practice Guideline (Columbia, MD: AMDA, 2010), 1–71.

22. E. Rachael, R.E. Bennett, M. Tuttle, K. May, J. Harvell, E.A. Coleman, "Health Information Exchange in Post-Acute and Long-Term Care Case Study Findings: Final Report," U.S. Department of Health and Human Services, Office of Disability, Aging and Long-Term Care Policy, Office of the Assistant Secretary for Planning and Evaluation, 2007, *http://aspe.hhs.gov/daltcp/reports/2007/HIEcase.pdf* (accessed May, 11, 2009).

23. See note 22 above.

24. K. Hyer, L. Brown, A. Berman, L. Polivka-West, "Establishing and Refining Hurricane Response Systems for Long-Term Care Facilities," *Health Affairs (Millwood)*, 25 (2006): w407–w411.

25. See note 2 above.

26. Medicare Payment Advisory Commission (MEDPAC), "Report to the Congress: Reforming the Delivery System," June, 2008, *www.medpac.gov/documents/jun08_entirereport.pdf*

27. J. Kautter, G. Pope, M. Trisolini, S. Grund, et al., "Medicare Physician Group Practice Demonstration Design: Quality and Efficiency Pay-for-Performance," *Health Care Financial Review*, 29 (2007): 15–29.

The Case for Improvement

Patients need to be in the driver's seat when it comes to managing their health. This is particularly true for the chronic care population. Although healthcare professionals certainly influence patient decisions, they are involved in a patient's care for relatively short periods of time, for example, during acute events like hospitalizations or outpatient interventions. Most of the time, patients or lay caregivers make decisions about how to take medications and when to follow up with physicians and determine the precise method for implementing medical orders. Therefore, it is in our patients' best interests to arm them with the knowledge and skills they need to effectively manage their healthcare issues.

Patient Compliance

The evidence is clear: patient adherence rates, particularly with medications, are low. The World Health Organization (WHO) estimates that as many as 50% of patients fail to take medications correctly.[1] A study commissioned in the United States by the National Community Pharmacists Organization showed that three out of four patients failed to take their medications as directed.[2] The problem is pervasive. Patients of all ages, genders, levels of education, and socio-economic status fail to comply with medication regimes.[3] Meanwhile, healthcare professionals struggle to understand patient compliance, or more accurately, the reasons for noncompliance.

Healthcare policy attempts to create a new vision and broad strategies. The National Council on Patient Information and Education (NCPIE) released a national education plan for improving patient adherence to prescribed medications. The following actions are included in the recommendations:

- The establishment of multidisciplinary Medication Education Teams, which recognize the patient as the center of the process

- The removal of government regulations that inhibit adherence to promotion programming

- The assessment of literacy and the implementation of intervention strategies[4]

The Agency for Healthcare Research and Quality (AHRQ) advocates that, "Questions are the Answer" in improving healthcare for consumers. The consumer section of their Web page lists the top 10 questions to ask when receiving healthcare and offers the consumer a tool for building a personal question list.[5]

Chronic Illness

Among all of the recommendations for improvement is the central theme of patient-centered care. Healthcare professionals need to reframe their assumptions about preparing patients for self-care. Patients must be well-prepared to take the lead once the formal clinical care process ends. They need to be armed with knowledge and proven techniques for managing their health. In addition, healthcare professionals should develop mechanisms for truly partnering with patients and their caregivers in the clinical care process.

This becomes even more important when the patient has chronic disease. A survey of chronically ill adults in eight countries conducted by Schoen and colleagues found some of the highest rates of foregoing care in the United States. Reasons cited include cost; coordination problems; and medical, medication, or lab errors. In fact, chronically ill adults in the US had the "highest rates of medical errors, care coordination problems and high out of pocket costs."[6]

The Chronic Care Model, developed by the MacColl Institute, "identifies the essential elements of a healthcare system that encourage high quality chronic disease care." These elements include the community, the healthcare system, self-management support, delivery system design, and decision support and clinical information systems. Each element includes evidence-based concepts that improve the chronic care process. Use of the model can "foster productive interactions between informed patients who take an active part in their care and providers with resources and expertise."[7]

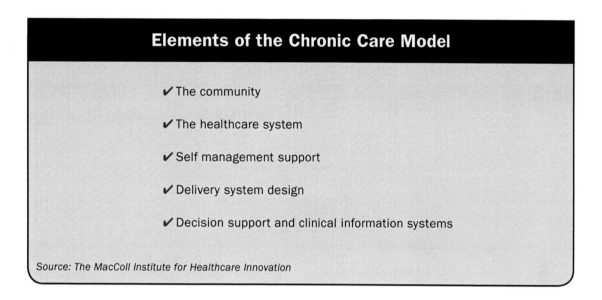

Elements of the Chronic Care Model

✔ The community

✔ The healthcare system

✔ Self management support

✔ Delivery system design

✔ Decision support and clinical information systems

Source: The MacColl Institute for Healthcare Innovation

A reactive health system

Researchers at McColl make the point that the health system as we know it is essentially reactive. Patients with chronic conditions need a healthcare delivery system that can anticipate clinical needs and prepare patients to manage them so they don't become crises. Further, clinicians need to rely on evidence-based guidelines and protocols in the treatment process. A consistent, overall approach based on best practice guidelines and collaboration by an interdisciplinary team of clinical professionals will benefit the patient in the long run. Because of this, a clinical information system that supports the clinical process of care and the team is essential. Complex patients with chronic diseases can't afford to have information fall through the cracks. Clinicians need to have information at their fingertips—information related both to the specific patient and to best practice guidelines.

A time investment

Probably the most significant challenge to our paradigms is the notion that patients need to be at the center of the care process and that healthcare professions need to collaborate with patients to design and implement care. This means that we can no longer spend 10 minutes giving the patient instructions or recommend that they attend a class. As Von Korff and colleagues found, patients and professionals need to work together to move through the entire care process, including establishing priorities, formulating goals, developing treatment plans, and making alterations based on a patient's response.[8] **Figure 2.1** depicts this essential concept.

Figure 2.1

Collaborative Chronic Care Process

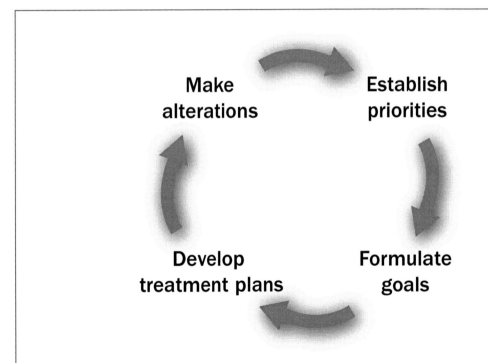

Adapted from: Patients and healthcare professionals working together in the clinical care process for managing chronic disease. Von Korff, Gruman, Schaefer, Curry, Wagner "Collaborative Management of Chronic Illness"

The Disease Management Association of America (DMAA) emphasizes patient self-management as central to chronic disease intervention. Healthcare professionals searching for optimal processes to support patient self-management may find the Outcomes Guideline Report assembled by The Care Continuum Alliance of the DMAA helpful.[9]

Patient self-management support was defined by the Institute of Medicine in 2003 as "the systematic provision of education and supportive interventions by healthcare staff to increase patients' skills and confidence in managing their health problems, including regular assessment of progress and problems, goal setting, and problem-solving support."[10] Patient management support programs that have been shown to be effective in improving outcomes and reducing utilization emphasize patient health literacy, knowledge of the healthcare system, and access of timely treatment.

Summary

As the population ages, chronic disease becomes more prevalent and requires us to alter traditional thinking about clinical care processes and patient involvement. Effective treatment includes partnering with patients and caregivers when moving through each component. On a strategic level, healthcare systems must be designed so the patient can participate actively in the chronic care process.

In the following chapters, we will describe some of the approaches that can be taken to work in partnership with patients and family caregivers to create and implement chronic care interventions, ultimately reducing the need for frequent, emergent trips to the hospital.

References

1. World Health Organization, *Adherence to Long-Term Therapies: Evidence for Action*. (World Health Organization, 2003).

2. National Community Pharmacists Association, "Take As Directed: A Prescription Not Followed," Research conducted by The Polling Company™. December 15, 2006.

3. L. Osterberg, T. Blaschke, "Drug Therapy: Adherence to Medication," *The New England Journal of Medicine*, 353 (2005): 487–97.

4. The National Council on Patient Information and Education, *Enhancing Prescription Medication Adherence: A National Action Plan* (Rockville, MD: NCPIE, 2007).

5. Agency for Healthcare Research and Quality, "Questions Are the Answer," *www.ahrq.gov/questionsaretheanswer/*.

6. C. Schoen, R. Osborn, S.K. How, M.M. Doty, J. Peugh, "In Chronic Condition: Experiences of Patients with Complex Healthcare Needs, in Eight Countries, 2008," *Health Affairs Web Exclusive*, (2008): w1–w16.

7. The Chronic Care Model. *www.improvingchroniccare.org/index.php?p=Model_Elements&s=18*. E.H. Wagner, B.T. Austin, C. Davis, M. Hindmarsh, J. Schaefer, A. Bonomi, "Improving Chronic Illness Care: Translating Evidence into Action," Health Affairs (Millwood), 20 (2001): 64–78.

8. M. Von Korff, J. Gruman, J.K. Schaefer, S.J. Curry, E.H. Wagner, "Collaborative Management of Chronic Illness," *Annals of Internal Medicine,* 127 (1997): 1097–1102.

9. Disease Management Association of America, *Care Continuum Alliance, Outcomes Guidelines Report, Volume 4* (Washington, DC: DMAA, 2009).

10. Institute of Medicine, *Priority Areas for National Action: Transforming Healthcare Quality* (Washington, DC: The National Academies Press, 2003), p. 52.

Patient Self-Management

LEARNING OBJECTIVES

After reading this chapter, you should be able to:

- Describe the characteristics of an adult-learning model

- Identify the levels of patient activation and the appropriate teaching methods associated with each

- Define literacy and health literacy and discuss the issues associated with low levels of both in the chronically ill adult population

Studies are beginning to show that patient self-management of chronic disease is effective in improving clinical outcomes and reducing utilization. Further, self-management strategies seem to be effective across all high volume conditions.[1-8] Krumholz and colleagues specified, in their randomized controlled study, the degree of improved resource utilization with patient education and support only. Patients with the high-volume chronic condition, congestive heart failure, experienced a 40% decrease in total readmissions, a 50% decrease in heart failure admissions, and a cost savings per patient of $7,515. These researchers showed patient self-management worked, even when provided without a medical management component.[9]

Some clinical research provides insight into how to best structure patient self-management support. Norris and colleagues assert that instructional programming involving patient collaboration may be more effective than a didactic approach.[10] In a follow-up study, Norris found that increasing educational contact time improved the effect of patient self-management education.[11] It seems taking time to engage patients in self-management education can pay off.

How Do Adults Learn?

In order to assist patients in managing their own health, it is important to understand how adults learn. The structure of most patient education provided in healthcare is based on methods used to teach healthcare professionals, which is based largely on pedagogical models. Although often used to describe the educational process in general, pedagogy literally means the art and science of teaching children. Pedagogical methods, for the most part, are teacher-directed methods. The teacher decides what should be learned, how it should be learned, when it will be learned, and, to a large degree, whether it is learned. In order to examine and analyze the patient education process, let's take a look at the experience of Mrs. B.

Mrs. B is a college-educated, 46-year-old woman who suffered a mild stroke. She seems to experience no ongoing effects. Because she is a single mother who provides the primary care for her young son with special needs, she is anxious to get home. Each day, she has been asking every member of the clinical team whether she could receive any necessary treatment at home. The cause of the stroke is unknown, and the decision is made to initiate ongoing treatment with anticoagulants. She leaves the hospital with an enoxaparin sodium (LOVENOX®) kit and instructions to administer this by injection until beginning therapy with warfarin (Coumadin, Jantoven). As Mrs. B is being discharged, a nurse visits her to teach her to administer an injection. While reviewing the discharge paperwork, the nurse reviews the materials in the kit and describes the procedure for self-administration of an injection. Mrs. B doesn't seem to be listening closely, but the nurse thinks this may be because Mrs. B self-administered injections when trying to become pregnant several years ago. The nurse follows her usual procedure for discharge teaching, covering everything on the checklist, and Mrs. B indicates she understands everything. It is almost time for the nurse to do her medication rounds, so she wraps up the teaching and recommends that Mrs. B call the cardiology clinic to receive education on warfarin therapy.

More effective patient education methods are based on an adult learning model (**Figure 3.1**). Malcolm Knowles outlines several assumptions that form the basis of adult learning:

1. **The Need to Know.** If adults perceive a need to learn something, they will be more motivated to learn it. Therefore, it is important for educators of adults to make them aware of how the learning will benefit them.

2. **The Learner's Self-Concept.** Adults, for the most part, are responsible for their own lives. They make their own decisions and are self-directed. However, in a learning situation, they often revert to the environment of childhood, which is that of a passive participant: tell me, teach me, and perhaps I will listen, but I might not do anything with all this information. Adult educators need to permit the learner to direct much of the learning process.

3. **The Role of the Learner's Experience.** Adults come to the learning experience with a great deal of prior knowledge and experiences. Let's face it: good or bad, patients have been making decisions about their health long before they had access to healthcare educators. They are not blank slates on which we can write the nascent rules of a healthy lifestyle. Some of the information we have decided they must learn may complement what they are already doing, but some of that information may contradict their long-held beliefs.

4. **Readiness to Learn.** Adults become ready to learn things that will help them cope with situations they are dealing with now. Patients may not be ready to learn about the long-term progression of their disease until it is upon them. They will be more ready to learn about the beginning stages while they are *in* the beginning stages. Learning will need to continue as the disease progresses.

5. **Orientation to Learning.** Adults are motivated to learn things that will help them solve problems in real life, rather than theoretical issues that they may never face. This has important implications for the materials used by patient educators. Those materials must be the same materials and cover the same information the patient will need to manage their own health.

6. **Motivation.** For the most part, adults are motivated by internal pressures, not external forces. Examples of internal motivators are the desire for improved quality of life, self-esteem, and satisfaction. Patient educators, no matter how zealous they are, cannot motivate an adult learner. The motivation must originate with the patient.[12]

Figure 3.1	

Assumptions of Adult Learning

The Need to Know	"How will learning this benefit me?"
The Learner's Self-Concept	"I will passively listen unless I am engaged as an active partner."
The Role of the Learner's Experience	"I know something about this. How does this new learning augment my existing knowledge base?"
Readiness to Learn	"How does this new information help me solve a problem I am facing now?"
Orientation to Learning	"I will learn more if I use the same tools in the learning environment as I will use in real life."
Motivation	"I want to learn this as much as you want me to learn it."

Carl Rogers defines the role of the adult educator as that of a facilitator of learning.[13] If the role of the patient educator is reframed as a facilitator of learning using an adult learning model, Mrs. B's experience would be quite different. The patient educator should assess Mrs. B's readiness to learn, her existing knowledge about her health, and what might be motivating her to make a change. Further, the nurse should present the information using the tools Mrs. B would actually use, and Mrs. B should try the skill for the first time as she is guided by the educator. With the adult learning concept in mind, let's take another look at Mrs. B's case.

Mrs. B had a child with special needs at home about whom she was very worried. Mrs. B had been quite assertive about her desire to be discharged soon after she arrived at the hospital. Though she didn't seem to be listening closely to the instruction, Mrs. B told the discharge nurse that she was confident in her ability to administer her injections correctly because she had done it a few times many years before while trying to become pregnant. If the discharge nurse really thought about this patient's readiness to learn, she probably would have concluded that Mrs. B simply wanted to get home to her child and therefore would indicate that she understood, even if she did not. Further, the education was probably not occurring at an optimal time for Mrs. B because her primary concern was getting home to her child; administering her injection would not have to be faced until the following day. The optimal time to facilitate learning and guide her through the process of administering the injection would have been at home the next day.

Since Mrs. B was college-educated, we can assume she has a self-concept supporting an educational process. In addition, she did have some experience with the self-administration of injections. The patient educator could have used that information to make Mrs. B an active participant in the process, either reinforcing good practices or correcting deficient ones. As most adults do, this learner had some experience on which to draw. An effective approach would have been to ask Mrs. B about the methods she had used. This would enable the patient educator to assess how much Mrs. B remembered and provide a foundation upon which she could build.

Once ready to receive the education related to the administration of the injection, the actual tools Mrs. B would be using should be available to guide her through the process. It would not be as effective to provide her with a theoretical description of how to administer an injection using a kit that may not resemble the one she actually receives from the pharmacy.

In this case, the discharging nurse did not attempt to discover what Mrs. B might already know about stroke or whether she might have the knowledge base or motivation to manage the ongoing treatment. Rather, the nurse simply referred Mrs. B to the cardiology clinic for further instruction. In following an adult learning model, a patient educator could have discussed the physiology of stroke and the benefits of ongoing prevention. Perhaps the greatest motivation for Mrs. B would be that she would continue to be able to care for her child; this discussion would not only make the benefit of following the treatment plan obvious, but would provide internal motivation for Mrs. B. Note the use of discussion as a teaching method here. The assumption is that Mrs. B would be an active participant, not a passive listener.

The timing of the educational process is an important consideration. To follow the adult education model, Mrs. B could not benefit from even the best process as she sits on the bed, dressed in her street clothes, ready to get in the wheelchair that will take her out the front door. Some of the education could have been facilitated early in the hospital stay, and some would have been best facilitated in her home, following the hospital stay.

Mrs. B—Patient Education Strategy

- **Readiness to learn:** Meet Mrs. B where she is. She needs to attend to her child before she will be ready to learn.

- **Learner's self-concept:** Mrs. B will respond positively if you involve her in the educational process. Make her an active partner.

- **Role of the learner's experience:** Mrs. B has some experience self-administering injections. Ask her to show you what she remembers and then guide her if she does something incorrectly.

- **Orientation to learning:** During the teaching, use the actual injection kit Mrs. B will be using at home.

- **Motivation:** A personal goal will often provide the patient with the motivation to learn. For Mrs. B, this might be retaining the ability to care for her son.

Get Ready for the Activated Patient

Patient education typically assumes that once provided with information, patients have the necessary ability to manage their health. This assumption suggests every patient has understood, agreed with, and internalized information related to his or her disease, its causes, and the patient's personal role in ongoing management. It also assumes all patients are functionally able to do what we ask of them; therefore, any patients who have difficulty in doing exactly what they have been told to do are labeled *noncompliant*.

As we learned in the last section, adults could be noncompliant because the education provided did not meet their needs as adult learners, or they simply lacked confidence that they can follow through. Hibbard and colleagues have shown patients have different levels of activation. Patient activation is defined as the patients' levels of knowledge, skill, and confidence regarding their own ability to manage their health and healthcare. Patients who lack knowledge, skill, and confidence are less activated and are therefore less able to perform the tasks required in managing their health.[14] Hibbard found that tailoring self-management education and support to a patient's level of activation was more effective than the usual disease management approach. Further, clinical indicators improved and utilization decreased.

The four levels of activation provide insight into attitudes, behaviors, and motivation that can impact a patient's ability to implement the behavior change necessary for self-management. Patients can move along a continuum of increasing levels of activation as they feel more able to take charge of their health. Similarly, patients can experience decreasing levels of activation when stress and other obstacles to self-management increase.

Level 1 activation—Starting to take a role

The patient does not feel confident enough to play an active role in his or her own health. Individuals at this level probably understand they are not following through on what they need to do to self-manage. However, they are not knowledgeable about their medical conditions or what they need to do in terms of self-care and may not understand they need to play an active role in managing their health. They tend to see themselves as passive recipients of care.[15]

Mrs. L is a 70-year-old, obese woman who was admitted to the hospital with pneumonia. She has a history of diabetes and her A1C level is 10.5%, indicating a glucose level that has been out of control for some time. While in the hospital, Mrs. L tells her nurse, "I am not a real diabetic because I don't take insulin." Despite receiving extensive diabetic teaching during her hospitalization, Mrs. L failed to test her glucose levels in the 72 hours following her discharge. When questioned by the nurse who visited her at home, Mrs. L explained, "Oh, I just haven't gotten around to that yet."

The goal of self-management education and support here is to enable Mrs. L to understand she has a critical role to play in becoming healthier. However, she may not yet have a need to know and the teaching techniques used thus far have probably required her only to listen without necessarily internalizing the information. This learner's self-concept has put her in a passive role.

Because Mrs. L has experienced a recent hospitalization, she may become ready to learn if the education and support provided could help her understand her role in the hospitalization and how critical it is. She may become engaged now to solve the problem she is currently experiencing. Consider asking, "What do you think caused your recent hospitalization?" A discussion about the relationship between infections and glucose levels could follow.

Mrs. L is just getting started on the path to activation, so it will be important not to overwhelm her, which could cause her to become frustrated and give up. It is important to take small steps and set her up for some amount of early success, motivating her to continue. Helping Mrs. L focus on one small step at a time, and giving her permission to put everything else on her long list of self-management tasks on hold for now, will help her feel less overwhelmed. The key is for her to start to experience some success with a small step. When the possibility of success is evident, there is an increase in motivation.

Mrs. L—Patient Education Strategy

- **Readiness to learn:** Mrs. L may be ready to learn because of her recent hospitalization, since this is generally a scary experience for patients. Help her understand how managing her diabetes can help her stay out of the hospital.

- **Set Mrs. L up for early success:** Start small with something she can realistically accomplish and build from there.

Level 2 activation—Building knowledge and confidence

Patients at this level have not had a great deal of success in attempts made to improve their health. In addition, they are not adequately knowledgeable about their medical issues. Therefore, they lack confidence in their ability to do anything about improving their health.

Mr. J told the nurse who visited him at home that, while in the hospital, he agreed to attend a diabetes class. However, he never really intended to follow through because, "I attended one of those after the last time I was in the hospital and it didn't do any good." Further discussion revealed Mr. J felt overwhelmed by the class and many of the materials provided; therefore, he left the session feeling that he could never accomplish all that was necessary to manage his diabetes successfully. Mr. J did not seem to retain much of what was taught in class, but he did remember that he was supposed to check his blood glucose levels every day. He just wasn't sure how to keep his blood glucose levels within an acceptable range.

Building confidence can lead to people being more open to learning. Learning can also lead to greater confidence. Because Mr. J did attend a class, the educator may be able to build upon anything he remembers and try to build his confidence in making another attempt at self-management. The education should build upon the learner's experience. Mr. J remembers the instruction regarding the testing; the patient educator could provide positive feedback on that and move from there to a discussion of decision-making, based on the information revealed in the testing. Begin with, "You have done a great job in testing your blood sugar levels daily. Let's talk about your diet next. What do you typically eat for breakfast? Lunch? Dinner? What about snacks?"

Because Mr. J expresses uncertainty about how to keep his blood glucose levels at an acceptable range, he may be motivated to learn. The educator can use that and his self-concept to encourage active participation.

Mr. J—Patient Education Strategy

- **Role of the learner's experience:** Because Mr. J attended a class and retained some information, use that to begin the educational process and engage him as an active participant in the learning process. Ask what he remembers and build from there.

- **Motivation:** Mr. J is beginning to ask questions so he may be motivated to learn more. Answer his questions to his satisfaction and build from there.

Level 3 activation—Taking action

At this level, patients are beginning to take some action to improve their health but may not have enough knowledge to be confident and consistent. Patients have a grasp of the main points but do not yet have the confidence and skill to actively manage their health.

Mrs. R had been a smoker since she was a teenager. She quit a year ago and, at age 69, seems to be committed to remaining smoke-free. She was aware of her history of chronic obstructive pulmonary disease (COPD) but thought that, because she quit smoking, her symptoms would diminish entirely without much more intervention on her part.

Mrs. R's successful attempt to quit smoking demonstrates that she is capable of making significant behavioral change to maintain her health. This success can lay the foundation for the work she must do to manage her COPD. Her knowledge and confidence can be improved by using her basic understanding of COPD and keeping in mind her success in achieving a difficult behavior change. Consider saying, "By quitting smoking, you have succeeded where most people fail. I am confident you can manage your COPD as well. So, let's talk about what you are doing now. How are you currently managing your symptoms?"

It is critical to use Mrs. R's experience as the foundation for her growth. In addition, remember that education will be much more effective if the educational process is oriented to the specific techniques and materials she will actually use in managing her COPD.

Mrs. R—Patient Education Strategy

- **The role of the learner's experience:** Mrs. R has succeeded in quitting smoking—something many people fail to achieve. Use this experience to express your confidence in her and build on it for future growth.

Level 4 activation—Maintaining behaviors

Patients at this level have made most of the behavior changes necessary to maintain their health and have a good understanding of their chronic disease. However, they may have difficulty in maintaining their healthy behaviors in times of stress.

Mr. S, a retired professor at a local university, thoroughly researched congestive heart failure when he was diagnosed and adheres to his cardiologist's instructions regarding diet, medication management, and follow-up testing—for the most part. His wife's health is failing and he is her primary caregiver. When he begins to feel overwhelmed by managing her medical issues, he forgoes dedication to his own regimen.

Mr. S is probably ready to learn how to maintain healthy behaviors, even when feeling overwhelmed. Consider asking Mr. S, "What do you think sometimes prevents you from maintaining your usual dedication to the management of your CHF?"

Because he generally manages his CHF well, it will be important to draw on his experience, permit him to identify the difficulties he is currently facing, and partner with him to facilitate further learning.

Mr. S—Patient Education Strategy

- **The role of the learner's experience and self-concept:** Because Mr. S is knowledgeable about CHF, ask him how he generally does things and build from there. Engage him as an active partner.

- **Resources:** Acknowledge Mr. S' stress and help him identify resources he can work with to develop an approach to manage his stress.

Hibbard and colleagues have developed the Patient Activation Measure, which is used to assess patients' activation and can be used to tailor self-management education. The assessment and educational materials are available through Insignia Health at *www.insigniahealth.com*.

What If Mr. Smith Can't Read?

The healthcare system runs on the written word. Most instructions, forms, prescriptions, and educational materials are provided to patients in writing. However, the U.S. Department of Education estimates that 14% of the adult population doesn't read well enough to understand a newspaper story written at an eighth-grade level.[16] Health literacy is a more pervasive problem. The Institute of Medicine estimates that nearly half of American adults have difficulty understanding and acting upon health information.[17] Even people with acceptable reading skills can have low levels of health literacy.

Literacy is defined as the ability to read, write, compute, and use technology at a level that enables an individual to reach his or her full potential as a parent, employee, and community member.[18] Health literacy includes the ability to access, understand, and apply basic health information (**Figure 3.2**). It includes the following abilities:

+ **Prose literacy**—the ability to understand and accurately use words

+ **Numeracy**—the ability to perform basic calculations

+ **Document literacy**—the ability to complete forms[19]

Figure 3.2

The Health Literacy Equation

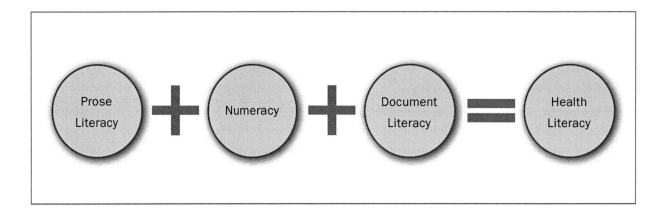

Inadequate health literacy is associated with poor health outcomes. These outcomes include increased incidence of chronic illness and related issues of poor health knowledge and low use of preventive health services.[20] Therefore, it is important to consider health literacy in any effort to improve patient self-management.

It is often difficult to tell whether a patient has inadequate levels of literacy or health literacy, especially during a four-day hospital stay or a 15-minute office visit. Individuals with limited literacy come from all walks of life. In fact, most individuals with limited literacy are Caucasian and use English as their primary language.[21] The level of formal education completed does not necessarily indicate limited literacy. Almost 25% of participants who scored at the lowest literacy level on the U.S. Department of Education's *National Adult Literacy Survey* were high school graduates.[22]

As anyone who has worked with limited-literacy patients knows, most have developed pretty successful strategies for hiding it. So assessing literacy would seem to be an important component of patient self-management education, yet it is not part of the traditional process. Perhaps that is because most assessments of literacy are awkward to incorporate into a medical environment. The two assessments most often used in healthcare research are the Test of Functional Health Literacy in Adults (TOFHLA) and the Rapid Estimate of Adult Literacy in Medicine (REALM). Both use lists of words that the patient is asked to read aloud. Neither uses medical terms, and neither numeracy nor document literacy are assessed.

Weiss and colleagues have developed a health literacy assessment test that can be incorporated into any patient self-management educational process. The test, called the *Newest Vital Sign*, is based on a nutrition label for ice cream. Its criterion validity correlates with the TOFHLA.[23]

The Newest Vital Sign requires three minutes to administer five or six questions, depending on patient responses. Because it uses a subject matter that could be part of any patient self-management educational process, this assessment can be incorporated as part of the natural flow of the process. It also spares patients the embarrassing experience of stumbling through lists of words before it finally becomes obvious they can't read.

Both the tool and a packet for implementation are available free of charge for healthcare professionals through *www.pfizerhealthliteracy.com.*

When working with patients with low health literacy, it is even more important not to overwhelm them and to use the adult learning model. To create a firm foundation on which to build, allow ample time to use the learner's experience and discover how the patient has been managing his or her health issues so far. Because formal educational experiences have probably not been positive, consider the patient's self-concept and encourage him or her to take an active role in the educational process.

Additionally, consider doing the following:

- **Limit the use of medical jargon and acronyms.** Patients may not know what "emesis" or "BID" means, for example. In addition, they may have something different in mind when the word *stool* is used.

- **Use illustrations to replace or enhance instructions and educational material.** Pictures help increase understanding of complex information for all patients.

- **Keep language simple and direct.** This is particularly difficult in conveying negative information, but patients cannot benefit from an attempt to ease the delivery of this kind of information if they cannot understand it.

- **Check for understanding.** Ask the patient to explain what he learned in his own words.

A Word About the Softer Side

My hope is that this chapter has helped you think differently about educating adults as they journey toward successful self-management. As you incorporate any of these tools into your educational process, it is important to remember to treat each patient with patience and respect. While we work with healthcare information every day, it is a new experience for most patients. Paradoxically, as adults, they will come to the learning experience with knowledge, beliefs, and biases that may enhance or hinder the process. It is important to recognize and use this dichotomy. It is also important to recognize that all of your nonverbal cues will either support or hinder the learning process. While we have talked a lot about creating an individualized educational process designed to meet the learner's needs, it cannot be overemphasized that most people respond positively to a learning environment that also feels supportive.

References

1. A. Warsi, P.S. Wang, M.P. LaValley, J. Avorn, D.H. Solomon, "Self-Management Education Programs in Chronic Disease: A Systematic Review and Methodological Critique of the Literature." *Archives of Internal Medicine*, 164(2004): 1641–1649.

2. J. Chodosh, S.C. Morton, W. Mojica, M. Maglione, M.J. Suttorp, L. Hilton, et al., "Meta-analysis: Chronic Disease Self-Management Programs for Older Adults." *Annals of Internal Medicine*, 143(2005): 427–438.

3. T. Effing, E.M. Monninkhof, P.P. van der Valk, G.G. Zielhuis, E.H. Walters, J.J. van der Palen, et al., "Self-Management Education for Patients with Chronic Obstructive Pulmonary Disease," *Cochrane Database of Systematic Reviews*, Issue 4. Art. No. (2007): CD002990. DOI: 10.1002/14651858.CD002990.pub2.

4. P.G. Gibson, H. Powell, J. Coughlan, et al., "Self-Management Education and Regular Practitioner Review for Adults with Asthma," *Cochrane Database Systematic Reviews,* 3 (2002): CD001117. DOI: 10.1002/14651858.CD001117

5. A.C. Faul, P.A. Yankeelov, N.L. Rowan, P. Gillette, L.D. Nicholas, K.W. Borders, et al., "Impact of Geriatric Assessment and Self-Management Support on Community-Dwelling Older Adults with Chronic Illnesses," *Journal of Gerontological Social Work*, 52(2009): 230–49.

6. U. Subramanian, F. Hopp, A. Mitchinson, J. Lowery, "Impact of Provider Self-Management Education, Patient Self-Efficacy, and Health Status on Patient Adherence in Heart Failure in a Veterans Administration Population," *Congestive Heart Fail*, 14(2008): 6–11.

7. P.G. Gibson, F.S. Ram, H. Powell, "Asthma Education," *Respiratory Medicine*, 97(2003): 1036–44.

8. A.A. Jonker, H.C. Comijs, K.C. Knipscheer, D.J. Deeg, "Promotion of Self-Management in Vulnerable Older People: A Narrative Literature Review of Outcomes of the Chronic Disease Self-Management Program (CDSMP)," *European Journal of Ageing*, 6(2009): 303–314.

9. Harlan M. Krumholz et al., "Randomized Trial of an Education and Support Intervention to Prevent Readmission of Patients with Heart Failure," *J Am Coll Cardiol*, 2002, 39: 83–89

10. S.L. Norris, M.M. Engelgau, K.M. Venkat Narayan, "Effectiveness of Self-Management Training in Type 2 Diabetes: A Systematic Review of Randomized Controlled Trials," *Diabetes Care*, 24(2001): 561–87.

11. S.L. Norris, J. Lau, S.J. Smith, et al., "Self-Management Education for Adults with Type 2 Diabetes: A Meta-analysis of the Effect on Glycemic Control," *Diabetes Care*, 25(2002): 1159–71.

12. Malcolm Knowles. *The Adult Learner: A Neglected Species* (Houston: Gulf Publishing Company, 1984), 52–61.

13. C.R. Rogers, *Freedom to Learn* (Columbus, Ohio: Charles Merrill, 1969), 104–105.

14. J.H. Hibbard, J. Greene, M. Tusler, "Improving the Outcomes of Disease Management by Tailoring Care to the Patient's Level of Activation," *Am J Manag Care*, 2009, 15(6): 353–361.

Chapter 3

15. Insignia Health, PAM Scoring and Interpretation, 2008.

16. U.S. Department of Education, National Center for Education Statistics, *National Assessment of Adult Literacy, 2003.*

17. Institute of Medicine, *Health Literacy: A Prescription to End Confusion* (Washington, DC: The National Academies Press, 2004).

18. ProLiteracy Worldwide, "Basic Facts about Literacy," *www.proliteracy.org/NetCommunity/Page.aspx?pid=345&srcid=191* (accessed February 14, 2010).

19. Pfizer Clear Health Communication Initiative, "What is Health Literacy?" *www.pfizerhealthliteracy.com/physicians-providers/newest-vital-sign.html* (Accessed February 21, 2010).

20. N.D. Berkman, D.A. DeWalt, M.P. Pignone, S.L. Sheridan, K.N. Lohr, L. Lux, et al., *Literacy and Health Outcomes. Evidence Report/Technology Assessment No. 87* (Prepared by RTI International–University of North Carolina Evidence-based Practice Center under Contract No. 290-02-0016), (AHRQ Publication No. 04-E007-2. Rockville, MD: Agency for Healthcare Research and Quality, 2004).

21. B.D. Weiss. "Epidemiology of Low Health Literacy," in *Understanding Health Literacy: Implications for Medicine and Public Health*, ed. J.G. Schwartzberg, J.B. VanGeest, C.C. Wang (Chicago: American Medical Association Press, 2005), 17–42.

22. I.S. Kirsch, A. Jungeblut, L. Jenkins, A. Kolstad, *Adult Literacy in America: A First Look at the Results of the National Adult Literacy Survey* (Washington, DC: National Center for Education Statistics. U.S. Department of Education, 1993).

23. B.D. Weiss, M.Z. Mays, W. Martz, K.M. Castro, D.A. DeWalt, M.P. Pignone, et al, "Quick Assessment of Literacy in Primary Care: The Newest Vital Sign," *Annals of Family Medicine*, 3 (2005): 514–522.

Reengineering the Hospital Discharge

LEARNING OBJECTIVES

After reading this chapter, you should be able to:

- Identify the most frequent adverse events that occur after a hospitalization and their causes.

- Describe the RED process, including its 11 components.

- Describe the roles of discharge advocate (DA) and embodied conversational agent (ECA).

Expectations for self-care after a hospitalization are becoming more challenging for patients. And, given shorter lengths of stay, the clinical team is pressured to prepare patients to perform more complex tasks than ever before, in a more concentrated timeline. Therefore, it makes sense to hone the discharge process to its most essential elements and perform the discharge tasks as efficiently and reliably as possible.

Numerous studies point to adverse events that occur all too frequently after discharge. In fact, Forster and colleagues found that 20% of discharges result in an adverse patient event.[1] The growth in the use of hospitalists has not been accompanied by concomitant development of processes for ensuring information exchange between physicians.[2] Moore and colleagues found that 30% of recommended post-discharge testing was not completed. Poor documentation in discharge summaries was cited as one cause.[3] Unfinished business seems to be another cause of post-discharge adverse events. Roy and his team found that 41% of inpatients were discharged with a pending test result, and over 9% may have required some action.[4] Patients experiencing some type of error related to post-discharge services were six times more likely to be re-hospitalized within three months. These factors lead to the revolving emergency room door too many patients experience.[5]

The Reengineered Discharge (RED)

The work accomplished by Dr. Brian Jack and colleagues seems to be timely. This team at Boston University's School of Medicine calls itself *Project RED* (reengineered discharge). They use engineering and quality improvement techniques to analyze the discharge process and recommend iterative changes in design.[6] The reengineered discharge process developed by this group uses a discharge advocate (DA) to coordinate all aspects of discharge and features a discharge checklist similar to those used by pilots to prepare for flights. Starting within 24 hours of admission to the hospital, discharge advocates meet with patients every day to provide education. On the day of discharge, the DA provides and reviews with the patients their spiral bound color-coded After Hospital Care Plan (AHCP). This booklet is used to reinforce patient teaching that has been done throughout the hospital stay regarding the patient's primary diagnosis, medications, and after-hospital care. Patients can benefit from additional teaching of the AHCP done by an "embodied conversational agent" (ECA) computer program run at the bedside on a kiosk. This discharge package can be used to educate all patients but is particularly useful for individuals with low health literacy.[7]

Principles of RED

Dr. Jack and his team developed RED based upon a few basic principles. Baseline analysis revealed there were many staff members involved in some aspects of the discharge process but no one who took charge of the entire process. So Dr. Jack and his team more clearly defined the roles involved. Because patients who have a clear understanding of their discharge instructions are 30% less likely to visit an emergency room or be readmitted to the hospital, patient education is provided during the hospitalization. Finally, given the importance of aftercare and physician follow-up, methods for ensuring communication with a patient's physician are emphasized.[8]

Operational Components of RED

There are 11 specific components included in the RED process that are mutually reinforcing. These are organized into the RED checklist that is used by DAs to ensure a consistent discharge process. We will review each component and discuss the role of the DA, embodied conversational agent (ECA), and clinical pharmacist in the process.

RED checklist

· Educate patients throughout the stay regarding their primary diagnosis and any relevant comorbidities.

· Reconcile the discharge plan with national guidelines and critical pathways.

· Confirm the medication plan.

· Make appointments for any necessary after-hospital testing and physician follow-up.

· Discuss tests completed in the hospital with the patient and explain who will follow up with the results.

· Organize necessary post-discharge services.

· Instruct the patient on what to do if a problem arises.

· Expedite the transfer of the discharge summary to physicians and other clinicians who will be providing after-hospital treatment and services.

· Check for patients' understanding by asking them to explain their discharge plan.

· Provide patients with their written discharge plan.

· Telephone patients after discharge to reinforce the discharge plan and assist in solving any problems.

A fundamental role of the DA is to educate patients throughout their stay regarding their diagnosis. Therefore, the DA must be thoroughly conversant in the patient's medical record and treatment plan, even before meeting with the patient. The DA is also responsible for reconciling the discharge plan with national guidelines and critical pathways. These plans and guidelines are reviewed with the medical team. The DA verifies the medications taken at home prior to hospitalization and confirms the medication plan. The DA also assists in reconciling the medication list developed on admission with the medications planned on discharge with the patient's team of physicians.[9] Let's follow Mrs. M and her DA, Sharon, an RN and former bedside nurse in a medical-surgical unit.

Mrs. M is a 75-year-old retired factory worker who is in the hospital with pneumonia. She has a history of COPD (related to her work environment), CHF, and knee replacement surgery. Our DA, Sharon, reviews the medical record, noting the names of the treatment team caring for Mrs. M. Sharon then contacts members of the treatment team to receive a complete description of the patient's diagnoses, medications, and treatment plan so she is familiar with each of these before meeting with Mrs. M. She also asks the team about the discharge plan for Mrs. M and compares it to national guidelines for pneumonia, Mrs. M's primary diagnosis. If there is a discrepancy between the national guidelines and the discharge plan proposed by the team, Sharon will attempt to resolve it before discharge by suggesting modifications to Mrs. M's discharge plan. Sharon will also verify the plan related to medications, as well as which medications will be discontinued, changed, and added. Sharon records all of the information she gathers into a data collection workbook so it can be incorporated into the after-hospital care plan (AHCP) that will be assembled for Mrs. M.[10]

Mrs. M—Discharge Advocate Strategies: Background

- Thoroughly familiarize yourself with Mrs. M's medical history and plan for this hospitalization.

- Compare the medical plan with national guidelines for Mrs. M's primary diagnosis. Resolve discrepancies.

Once the background information is assembled and the DA confirms the discharge plan with the medical team, it is time to meet with the patient. During this meeting, the DA will educate the patient regarding her primary diagnosis and any relevant comorbidities that are of concern to the patient. The patient will be asked to verbalize the details of the discharge plan to check for understanding. The DA will also discuss planned treatments, tests and procedures and make sure the patient knows who will give her results of tests or procedures and, if necessary, how to follow up and where to follow up. The medication list is reviewed with the patient, emphasizing each medication's purpose, side effects and correct administration. In addition, the DA will make sure the patient is able to obtain her medications. The DA also ensures the patient knows what to expect after discharge. The importance of keeping follow-up appointments is emphasized, and the DA organizes the discharge services, including clinician follow-up and post-discharge testing, according to the patient's preferences. Finally, the procedure for handling unanticipated problems is reviewed with the patient.[11] Let's check in with Sharon and Mrs. M.

Sharon meets with Mrs. M in her hospital room and begins the discussion by explaining her role as a discharge advocate. She then asks Mrs. M to explain why she has been hospitalized. In this way, Sharon can assess how much is already understood and utilize Mrs. M's experience to build a more complete understanding. Sharon encourages Mrs. M to ask questions and to stop her if she uses medical terms that are unfamiliar. When explaining Mrs. M's diagnosis, Sharon uses hospital-approved handouts that include information and illustrations. Because Mrs. M has indicated that she would like to learn more about pneumonia, Sharon leaves the information with her to review and take home. Sharon then asks Mrs. M about any other medical conditions she has. They talk about COPD and CHF and how those conditions relate to Mrs. M's primary diagnosis.

Sharon then talks with Mrs. M about the follow-up appointments she will require after the hospitalization. The hospitalist would like Mrs. M to follow up with her primary care physician (PCP) and a pulmonologist. Sharon asks Mrs. M whether there are any times or days she is not able to make it to an appointment and inquires about how she will get to her appointments. Mrs. M's daughter will transport her, so Sharon notes that Mrs. M will not need assistance in getting to her appointments and that the earliest she can make it to her appointments is

9:00 a.m. Once Sharon has made all of the follow-up appointments, she will visit Mrs. M again to confirm she will be able to keep the appointments that have been scheduled.

The next topic is medications. Sharon begins by asking Mrs. M whether she has any allergies. Since Mrs. M is allergic to sulfadiazine, Sharon ensures this has been recorded in the chart and Mrs. M is not being sent home on it. Sharon then asks about the presentation of the allergy and makes sure Mrs. M knows she should avoid this medication.

To ensure Mrs. M can obtain her discharge medications, Sharon asks about any potential problems. Sharon makes sure Mrs. M has a pharmacy and can get there to pick up her medications. Sharon also inquires about any other difficulties related to obtaining medications. Mrs. M tells Sharon that her pharmacy delivers, so Sharon will make sure prescriptions are faxed directly to the pharmacy upon discharge.

The next step is to reconcile the medications Mrs. M will need to continue at home with medications she was taking before her hospital admission. Sharon discusses with Mrs. M the list of medications developed on admission and asks her to verify what medications she was taking at home before her admission to the hospital. Mrs. M verifies that the listing is complete. So using the list provided by the treatment team, Sharon identifies the medications Mrs. M will no longer need to take after this hospitalization. Sharon also identifies new medications the medical team wants Mrs. M to take when she gets home.

Sharon then reviews all of the medications the treatment team wants Mrs. M to take when she gets home. Using the AHCP, Sharon goes through each medication, drawing Mrs. M's attention to the name of the medicine, the reason for the medicine, the number of pills to take, and what time of day she should take it. Sharon also discusses side effects Mrs. M should report to her PCP.

Since Mrs. M is going home on a low-sodium diet, Sharon calls that to Mrs. M's attention and asks if she understands how to follow the diet. Sharon also asks whether Mrs. M would like to discuss how to follow the diet with a nutritionist, either in the hospital or after she returns home. Finally, Sharon makes sure Mrs. M won't have difficulty obtaining low-sodium foods when she gets home.

Mrs. M's doctor has recommended physical therapy after the hospitalization so Sharon makes sure she knows why the therapy has been ordered and how important it is to complete. Sharon also discusses any suggestions or restrictions Mrs. M's doctor has made regarding physical exercise after the hospitalization.

Mrs. M is going home on oxygen, so Sharon makes sure she knows what it is for and how it will be delivered, and provides Mrs. M with a contact number should any problems arise with her oxygen delivery. To assist in clarifying this information for the patient regarding physical therapy and home oxygen, Sharon refers to the electronic medical record and contacts the case manager involved in setting up these patient services.[12]

Mrs. M—Discharge Advocate Strategies: Initial Meeting with the Patient

- Familiarize the patient with your role on the medical team.

- Use the learner's experience: Ask Mrs. M to explain why she has been hospitalized. Build your teaching from what she already knows. Use the learner's self-concept: this will encourage Mrs. M to be an active participant.

- Explain the purpose of follow-up appointments and negotiate the scheduling with Mrs. M.

- Reconcile medications, and ensure that Mrs. M understands how to take each medication and can obtain them after discharge.

- Educate Mrs. M on her diet and verify that she can follow it at home.

- Explain after-hospital services, emphasizing the contribution of these services to Mrs. M's recovery. Explain what to do if services do not arrive when expected.

On the day of discharge, all of the information that has been reviewed with the patient throughout her hospitalization is put into a written discharge plan in the form of the AHCP and is provided to the patient. The AHCP contains:

+ A description of the primary diagnosis.

+ Specific information on the discharge medications, including the names of all the medications, how to take them, the reason for each medication, and where to obtain them.

+ Information on symptoms to watch for and instructions on what to do if the condition deteriorates.

+ An organized listing of follow-up appointments for clinical visits and post-discharge testing.

+ A calendar page with the appointments and tests list.

+ Identification of test results not available at discharge and instructions regarding how to follow up on results.[13]

Sharon reviews all of Mrs. M's medications. Using the AHCP, Sharon goes through each medication, including any accompanying photographs, drawing Mrs. M's attention to the recommended dose and how often she should plan to take it. Sharon also discusses side effects Mrs. M should report to her PCP. Using the "teach back" technique, Sharon then asks Mrs. M to explain what she understands in her own words.

Sharon provides Mrs. M with a chart, which illustrates how Mrs. M should take her medications and reviews it with her. Sharon then tells Mrs. M that a pharmacist will call her in two or three days to make sure she understands any new medications, as well as any changes that may have been made to previous medications she was taking at home.

Sharon also explains each appointment with Mrs. M, explaining the reason for the appointment and reinforcing the location, date, and time. Sharon emphasizes the importance of bringing the AHCP to each of these appointments.

Mrs. M has some pending lab tests, and the results may not be available until after discharge. So Sharon identifies these tests for Mrs. M and emphasizes the importance of discussing these pending results with her PCP, who will receive the reports.

Sharon reviews potential problems that may occur once Mrs. M returns home. These generally relate to new medication side effects, difficulty acquiring medications, and clinical deterioration. Finally, Sharon provides Mrs. M with contact information for her PCP and DA so Mrs. M can call if she thinks of any questions or encounters any difficulties after returning home. This information is also clearly documented on Mrs. M's AHCP.

Sharon completes the in-hospital portion of the RED discharge after all components of the RED checklist are done. She completes patient teaching and ensures Mrs. M has a comprehensive understanding of her AHCP. Sharon documents any remaining notes or progress in a data collection workbook to allow communication to other team members regarding Mrs. M's discharge care.[14]

Mrs. M—Discharge Advocate Strategies: Day of Discharge

- Review all of Mrs. M's medications and ask her to explain the plan in her own words.

- Confirm the details of the after-hospital appointments and remind Mrs. M to bring her AHCP.

- Identify testing that will need to be completed after discharge and emphasize discussing these results with the physician who will be following Mrs. M after discharge.

- Review potential problems that may occur and ensure Mrs. M knows what to do.

Finally, within 48 hours of the patient's discharge, the DA expedites transmission of the discharge summary and patient's AHCP to the PCP. The discharge summary should include the following elements:

+ Identification of the principle diagnosis, along with a brief discussion of the reason for hospitalization

+ Enumeration of the significant findings, including the most recent reports for lab results, operative reports, and medication administration documentation

+ A listing of the procedures performed and related care, treatment, and services provided

+ Description of the patient's condition at discharge

+ A reconciled medication list, including allergies

+ Identification of acute medical issues and pending test results that require follow-up

+ Input from consultative services, including rehabilitative therapy

The last of the checklist components occurs two to three days after discharge. A clinical pharmacist telephones the patient to check on the patient's health status, reinforce the discharge medication plan, review appointments and any home health services, and remind the patient about what to do if a problem arises.[15]

Having access to Mrs. M's discharge summary and AHCP will familiarize the clinical pharmacist with her hospital stay and discharge plan.[16]

The discharge advocate

As defined in Dr. Jack's Training Manual, the role of the DA includes:

+ Coordinating with the medical team, RNs, and case managers

+ Educating patients about their disease

+ Educating patients about their medication(s)

+ Arranging aftercare with patients and family

+ Reinforcing national quality guidelines

+ Arranging for medication pick-up, rides

+ Preparing and reinforcing AHCP with patients and family[17]

In addition, the DA must possess the following qualities:

+ Excellent communication and education skills

+ The ability to establish a trusting relationship with patients, because a patient must feel comfortable to express doubts regarding self-care abilities or difficulties on following the discharge plan

+ Strong organization and multitasking skills, because patients in the caseload will not all be at the same point in the process, and the intervention will not be completed in its entirely in one sitting

+ The ability to earn the respect of the treatment team so they work with the DA and take her suggestions seriously

The embodied conversational agent

Dr. Jack and his team have also designed a computerized "embodied conversational agent" (ECA), named Louise, that assists the DA in delivering patient education and takes the patient through the AHCP. Patients follow a copy of their AHCP as Louise explains it. Using a touch screen, patients can ask Louise to repeat information, slow down, or stop for a while if they need to rest. The Project RED team designed Louise to mimic live clinicians explaining written medical instructions. Louise's explanations are supported by the colored illustrations in the AHCP. Dr. Jack and his associates estimate that it takes the DA 81 minutes to complete the total intervention with the patient. The computerized ECA can reduce that time by 30 minutes. In addition, 74% of patients in a pilot study preferred working with the ECA.[18]

The ECA is particularly helpful for patients with low health literacy levels. Because patients can direct the pace of information presented and repeat any part of the education, it enables patients to receive information in a time frame that is comfortable for them and not based upon the time available by the nurse. The computerized process delivers information the patient is ready to learn. Moreover, it encourages patients to be an active participant. Learners who have a self-concept that encourages more of a passive role related to educational processes will be nudged into a more active role.

Implementing RED

The RED program is dependent upon a treatment team that communicates and works together very effectively. Teams that do not share information regarding decisions affecting discharge will have a difficult time implementing RED. Therefore, when contemplating the implementation of RED, teams should set themselves up for success. Consider selecting one clinical team to pilot the program, taking note of successes and challenges so that learning and continuous improvement can be part of the process. The clinical team selected should be coalesced and have a strong organizational leader who can drive the implementation.

It would also be helpful to have a strong physician champion who can encourage other physicians on the team to communicate the discharge timing and needs as early in the process as possible. It is also critical for the physicians on the team to be supportive of this new process with their patients and take an active role in developing the discharge education. If implementing some of the information systems, it will be important to involve the information management department early so the computer system supports the new process. As your discharge process is being reengineered, it is important to make note of suggestions for improvement from the team. Team members will be more supportive of a process they helped to build. And finally, share the improved outcomes that will occur. Every team wants to know that the hard work has paid off.

Your proven success will help you move from the pilot phase to hospitalwide implementation.

Expected Outcomes

Carolyn M. Clancy, in her commentary in the *American Journal of Medical Quality*, identifies the major outcomes that resulted from the original work on RED. The fundamental outcome resulting from improved patient understanding of discharge information is a reduction in 30-day readmission rates. In fact, Dr. Jack's research shows more informed patients are 30% less likely to return to the hospital or visit the emergency department within 30 days. Patients who have the benefit of this process are also more likely to have a follow-up appointment with their PCP, and 91% of those physicians had the discharge summary within one day of the hospitalization. Not surprisingly, more than half of the patients in Dr. Jack's seminal work had medication problems that needed corrective action by the clinical pharmacist upon their arrival home. When asked 30 days after discharge about the experience, patients reported they felt more prepared for discharge after participation in RED. RED appears to be related to cost savings as well. After accounting for nursing time, RED saved $380 per patient.[19]

Where to Learn More

Dr. Jack and his team have developed a useful website that includes detailed descriptions of RED, a training manual for the DA, and videos from Louise, the ECA. Access *www.bu.edu/fammed/projectred/index.html* for more information.

References

1. A.J. Forster, H.J. Murff, J.F. Peterson, T.K. Gandhi, D.W. Bates, "The Incidence and Severity of Adverse Events Affecting Patients after Discharge from the Hospital," *Annals of nternal Medicine*, 138 (2003): 161–7.

2. R.M. Wachter, "Hospitalists in the United States—Mission Accomplished or Work in Progress?" *New England Journal of Medicine*, 350 (2004): 1935–6.

3. C. Moore, T. McGinn, E. Halm, "Tying Up Loose Ends: Discharging Patients with Unresolved Medical Issues," *Archives of Internal Medicine,* 167 (2007): 1305–11.

4. C.L. Roy, E.G. Poon, A.S. Karson, Z. Ladak-Merchant, R.E. Johnson, S.M. Maviglia, T.K. Gandhi, "Patient Safety Concerns Arising from Test Results that Return after Hospital Discharge," *Annals of Internal Medicine,* 143(2005): 121–8.

5. C. Moore, J. Wisnivesky, S. Williams, et al., "Medical Errors Related to Discontinuity of Care from an Inpatient to an Outpatient Setting," *Journal of General Internal Medicine*, 18(2): 646–51.

6. B.W. Jack, V.K. Chetty, J.L. Greenwald, G.M. Sanchez, A.E. Johnson, S.R. Forsythe, et al., "A Reengineered Hospital Discharge Program to Decrease Rehospitalization: A Randomized Trial," *Annals of Internal Medicine*, 150(2009): 178–87.

7. Project RED (Re-engineered Discharge), A Research Group at Boston University Medical Center, *www.bu.edu/fammed/projectred*, (Accessed April 3, 2010).

8. C.M. Clancy, "Reengineering Hospital Discharge: A Protocol to Improve Patient Safety, Reduce Costs, and Boost Patient Satisfaction," *Am J Med Qual*, 2009, 24: 344–346.

9. See note 6 above.

10. Brian W. Jack et al., "Final Training Manual," *www.bu.edu/fammed/forms/projectred/* (accessed April 4, 2010).

11. See note 6 above.

12. B.W. Jack, et al., "Final Training Manual," *www.bu.edu/fammed/forms/projectred/* (accessed April 10, 2010).

13. See note 6 above.

14. B.W. Jack et al., "Final Training Manual," *www.bu.edu/fammed/forms/projectred/* (accessed April 10, 2010).

15. See note 6 above.

16. B.W. Jack et al., "Final Training Manual," *www.bu.edu/fammed/forms/projectred/* (accessed April 10, 2010).

17. B.W. Jack et al., "Final Training Manual," *www.bu.edu/fammed/forms/projectred/* (accessed April 4, 2010).

18. B.W. Jack et al., "Louise: Saving Lives, Cutting Costs in Healthcare," Project RED: A Research Group at Boston University Medical Center *www.bu.edu/fammed/projectred/publications/VirtualPatientAdvocateWebsiteInfo2.pdf* (Accessed April 8, 2010).

19. See note 8 above.

Transitions Programming

The transitional period between levels of care can be fraught with uncertainty and complexity for patients, especially those trying to manage chronic disease. It is why so many return to hospitals with potentially preventable readmissions. If you imagine a relay race as an analogy to the healthcare process for this patient population, each provider's responsibility ends with a discharge—but the next provider doesn't pick up the baton right away. There is a period when the patient, and perhaps a friend or family caregiver, is left to run the race the best he can.

If managed appropriately, the transitional period can be an opportunity to prepare patient learners to self-manage. An acute episode that causes the patient to access care can certainly inspire the need to know. Most patients are motivated to make changes in their health following an acute illness. The key to long-term success can be maintaining that desire once the patient begins to feel better. Clinicians can make the best use of this transitional period by capitalizing on the patient's readiness to learn information they have a need for in this transitional period. Further, this period can be the ideal time to build on the patient's experience.

Two programs, developed by long-standing researchers and clinicians in this field, have successfully prepared patients to assume the baton and become a full participant in the race. Although there are many types of transitions in the healthcare system, both programs treat hospital admission and readmission as significant events that indicate patients are in need of intervention. Therefore, both programs focus a great deal of attention on the hospital admission as the starting place in the intervention, although these programs can augment a variety of healthcare transitions.

The Care Transitions Intervention[SM]—Eric A. Coleman, MD, MPH

The Care Transitions Intervention[SM] is an evidence-based, self-management model. It is led by Dr. Eric Coleman and is based on four conceptual domains that patients and caregivers have identified as the most important aspects of care.

These domains, referred to as "pillars," (**Figure 5.1**) include:

- Medication self-management

- A patient-centered record

- Primary care and specialist follow-up

- Knowledge of red flags warning symptoms or signs indicative of a worsening condition, and how to respond[1]

Figure 5.1

Care Transition Intervention Pillars

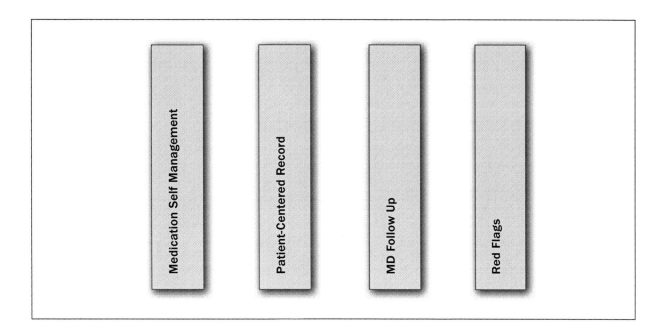

The transition coach

As explained in the Care Transitions Intervention[SM] Protocol Manual Version 2.0:

> *The transition coach is fundamental to encouraging the patient and family caregiver to assume a more active role in their care. Transition coaches do not fix problems and they do not provide skilled care. Rather, they model and facilitate new behaviors and communication skills for patients and families to feel confident in their ability to respond successfully to common problems that arise during care transitions. Thus, in the role of patient empowerment facilitator, the transition coach provides information and guidance to the patient and/or family for an effective care transition, improved self-management skills, and enhanced patient-practitioner communication.*

The transition coach typically begins working with a patient during a hospitalization and endeavors to visit patients early in their stay. There is also one home visit, typically within two days of discharge, and three follow-up phone calls.

Early in the relationship, the transition coach will work with the patient to establish a personal goal. This may be something the patient would like to do but has not yet been able to because of his or her health. Establishing this goal provides the motivation to self-manage.[2]

The key to successful transition coaching is to provide the patient with the specific tools and practice to self-manage once the transition coach is no longer involved. It sounds easy, but it takes new coaches time, practice, and focused feedback to move from their prior roles as *doers* into the coaching role. As we review the pillars, we will also discuss the role of the transition coach in order to see specifically what this role entails.

Medication self-management

Medications are often the biggest source of frustration for patients. As a result, many patients are simply not taking them. The World Health Organization has estimated that 50% of patients fail to take their medications as prescribed. The consequences are serious. Medication nonadherence leads to unnecessary progression of disease and complications, loss of functional ability, diminishing quality of life, and, in some instances, premature death.

The National Council on Patient Information and Education (NCPIE) has summarized the research findings associated with the reasons for patient nonadherence including those related to the medication, patient, prescriber, and pharmacy. Perhaps the largest obstacle is the complexity of the medication regimens. As the number of medications and dosing frequencies increase, adherence rates decrease. Side effects are another medication-related cause of medication nonadherence.

The greatest patient-related difficulties are simple forgetfulness and the inability to understand and act on the medication instructions. The latter is affected by high health literacy rates. Patients who do not understand the medications, why those medications are prescribed, and how they work may simply make a conscious choice not to take them. A significant number of patients do not make the connection between the health-related decisions they make and their poor health status.

The NCPIE found that a major factor related to patient nonadherence is the lack of physician awareness related to compliance management. Most physicians tend to overestimate their patients' ability to manage medications and the actual adherence level. Perhaps this contributes to the pervasive problem of poor communication between physicians and patients, including the lack of medication education that is provided to patients. Insufficient time and the lack of reimbursement for educational activities have also been cited as reasons for poor medication instruction.

Because of the frequency of contact between patients and pharmacists, the pharmacist has been identified as having great potential to influence medication adherence. However, issues related to time and privacy have been raised. Further, there is discussion among the professional community of pharmacists related to their role in medication education and the resources necessary to provide it.[3]

The goal of the Care Transitions Intervention Medication Self-Management pillar is: *The patient is knowledgeable about his medications and has a medication management system that works for him.* The transition coach asks the patient to show her what he takes and how he takes it. The patient then records what he is actually taking in the personal health record (PHR). The transition coach helps the patient identify any medication discrepancies and records questions for his doctor to resolve these discrepancies. We'll go through each of the Care Transitions pillars with Mr. D and his transition coach, an RN with hospital and home care experience.[4]

Mr. D is a 71-year-old patient who was hospitalized with an exacerbation of heart failure. His transition coach, Diane, begins working with Mr. D in the hospital, helping him establish a goal of walking through the neighborhood again. Although Mr. D is not knowledgeable about his health issues, he does not have serious literacy issues that need attention. Mr. D and Diane's work related to the medication pillar begins in the hospital. They begin exploring Mr. D's knowledge of his medications.

Diane visits Mr. D at home the day after discharge to facilitate reconciliation of his medications and help him identify any medication discrepancies. Mr. D's cardiologist ordered a change in his dose of lisinopril, but Mr. D has been taking the old dose. In addition, Mr. D takes a baby aspirin, but has just been put on warfarin therapy. He didn't think he needed to tell anyone in the hospital about the medications he takes without a prescription. Diane and Mr. D review the discharge instructions related to medications, and Diane watches Mr. D list in his PHR the medication he is taking. During this exercise, Mr. D has many questions related to dosing and side effects. He records these questions for his doctor in his PHR.

As Mr. D retrieves the medication bottles in order to make his list, Diane notices that he follows a complex system involving rubber-banding groupings of bottles for the medications he takes at the same time. He seems to run into trouble with this method once he encounters medications he needs to take more than once a day. Diane asks him if he would like to try a pill box. Mr. D says yes, and together they fill it for the week during the coaching visit. Diane also notices that Mr. D has a medication he took briefly for pain and never finished. It had expired. Diane and Mr. D discuss how he might dispose of it.

Diane makes three follow-up phone calls to Mr. D, during which she asks him questions related to his progress toward his personal goal and things they had discussed during the home visit, such as how the new medication system was working for him and the lab tests he planned to have. In this way, Diane can help celebrate his successes and be a resource for any challenges he is having related to medication management.

Mr. D—Medication Management Patient Coaching Strategy

- Assess Mr. D's knowledge and medication management system.

- Identify medication discrepancies after discharge.

- Organize a medication management system (if none exists).

- List medication questions for the follow-up physician visit.

- Continue to reinforce the medication system and answer any questions during the phone visits.

A patient-centered record

The goal for using the patient-centered record, the PHR, is that *the patient understands and uses it to facilitate communication and ensure continuity of the care plan across providers and settings.* It is a living document that is managed by the patient or by the informal caregiver. The following aspects are included in the record:

- The patient's health conditions in his own words

- Medications and allergies

- Advance care directives

- Warning symptoms or signs that correspond to the patient's chronic illness(es)

- Space for the patient and/or caregiver to record any questions and concerns in preparation for the next encounter

The PHR is intended to be maintained and updated by the patient or caregiver and shared with each practitioner at every visit.[5] Let's see how Mr. D and Diane address the patient-centered record at each of their visits.

Diane provides Mr. D with a PHR booklet during a hospital visit. She reviews the purpose and draws his attention to the listing of activities that should be completed before he leaves the hospital. She then asks him to complete as much of the record as he can. She encourages him to discuss questions or concerns with any of the clinicians who see him in the hospital.

During the home visit, Diane goes through the PHR with Mr. D as they discuss his personal goal and each of the four pillars. She then encourages Mr. D to take the PHR with him to his first physician visit following the hospitalization and every subsequent medical encounter.

When Diane follows up with Mr. D by phone, she asks about the outcome of physician visits or other medical appointments. She also asks whether Mr. D has updated his PHR and encourages him to continue using it.

Mr. D—Patient-Centered Record Coaching Strategies

> - Explain how to use the PHR.
>
> - Emphasize the importance of keeping the PHR updated and bringing it to all medical visits.
>
> - Establish and record a personal goal that is important to Mr. D.

Primary care and specialist follow-up

Jenks and colleagues reviewed rehospitalizations for Medicare patients and found that 50% of the patients readmitted within 30 days did not see a physician at any time during that period.[6] Completing follow-up appointments with a physician is an important factor in preventing a rehospitalization.

The goal for primary care and specialist follow-up is that *the patient schedules and completes a follow-up visit with the primary care physician (PCP) or specialist and is prepared to be an active participant in these interactions.* During the hospitalization, the transition coach discusses the importance of follow-up appointments with the specialist or the PCP.

During the home visit, the transition coach will assist the patient in prioritizing questions to ask related to medications, new health concerns, and future planning. The coach and patient may even role-play the discussion. Phone visits will be used to elicit feedback on the physician visit and strategize about how to get any remaining questions or concerns addressed.[7] Let's check in with Mr. D and see how he and Diane have handled this pillar.

During the hospital visit, Mr. D mentions that he plans to see his cardiologist for an office visit. Diane discusses this with Mr. D and asks him what he would like to accomplish during the visit. When Diane visits Mr. D at home, she is gratified to learn he did call his cardiologist to make an appointment. However, the secretary in the office gave him an appointment for three weeks later. Diane worked with Mr. D to develop a strategy for getting an earlier appointment. Mr. D phoned the office again while Diane was at his house so she could provide coaching and support, where necessary. He was able to get an appointment the next week. Diane and Mr. D developed a plan for the visit, which included bringing medications, using his PHR, and getting his three most important questions answered.

During the next phone visit, Diane asked Mr. D. how the doctor visit went. He was pleased with the amount of information he received and felt like a more active part of the process.

Mr. D—Physician Follow-up Coaching Strategies

- Develop an approach to secure a timely appointment.

- Organize information and questions for a productive visit.

- Prepare Mr. D to be an active participant.

Knowledge of Red Flags

The Institute of Medicine, in its *Healthy People 2010* report, reviewed the conceptual framework around the medical concept of prevention. Primary, secondary, and tertiary prevention can be expressed in terms that patients can readily understand (**Figure 5.2**). These include:

- **Primary Prevention**—How can I keep myself well?

- **Secondary Prevention**—If I am getting sick, how can I detect a problem early and get help quickly?

- **Tertiary Prevention**—If I am sick, how can I get the best medical care?[8]

Figure 5.2	
	Patients' Role in Prevention

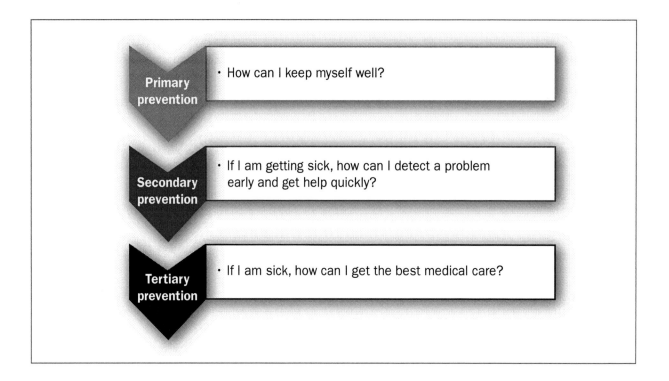

The goal of the Red Flags pillar is to *ensure the patient is knowledgeable about indicators that his or her condition is worsening and demonstrates knowledge of how to respond.*[9]

Diane gives Mr. D a teaching tool about heart failure, which includes an action plan, while he is in the hospital. During the hospital visit, Diane asks Mr. D to identify the symptoms that brought him to the hospital. Mr. D mentions shortness of breath and weight gain and remarks that he had been experiencing the symptoms for quite a while, but never attributed these symptoms to his congestive heart failure. Mr. D feels like he will be able to recognize the symptoms much earlier after his discussion with Diane.

When visiting Mr. D at home, Diane asks Mr. D how he is doing. He shows her his red flags tool and explains how he would access care if he experiences symptoms.

Mr. D—Red Flags Coaching Strategies

- Facilitate a discussion of signs and symptoms.

- Identify those the patient experienced.

- Practice the actions and role play, if appropriate.

Transitional Care—Mary Naylor, PhD, RN, FAAN

The Transitional Care Model, developed by Mary Naylor at the University of Pennsylvania, is another evidence-based intervention targeted toward chronically ill adults with complex medical needs. It emphasizes maximization of self-management and uses a transitional care nurse. As with the Care Transitions Program, this model begins with the hospitalization.

Master's-prepared, the advanced practice transitional care nurse acts as the primary coordinator of care across the entire episode of care, including the hospital stay. Guided by evidence-based protocols, the transitional care nurse provides comprehensive in-hospital planning, which includes patient education and recommendations for care modifications in collaboration with a multidisciplinary team. Within 24 hours of enrollment into the program, the transitional care nurse conducts a comprehensive assessment in order to obtain a beginning functional status and establish priority needs for the patient's stay.[10]

A home visit occurs within 24 to 48 hours of discharge. Once home, the transitional care nurse clarifies the discharge summary, reconciles medications, and works to ensure physician follow-up. As in the hospital, the transitional care nurse may make recommendations to the physician for modifications to the care plan. For example, once an assessment of the medication management system, including ability to obtain refills, is made, the transitional care nurse may recommend changes based on family finances and insurance coverage. During the first month, home visits occur once a week, followed by semi-monthly visits for the remainder of the program.

The transitional care nurse also accompanies the patient to the first follow-up visit with the physician and other physician visits, if necessary. The goal for the first visit is to facilitate understanding of the hospital discharge plan. The transitional care nurse directly facilitates and advocates on behalf of the patient. Overall, the transitional care nurse supports patients as they endeavor to have their concerns addressed and understand the physician's instructions.

There is emphasis on educating patients toward self-management. Patients are educated regarding warning signs, medication management, and physician orders. The transitional care nurse may facilitate referrals to Assisted Living, Chronic Case Management, or Palliative Care, as needed by the patient. The typical intervention is one to three months in duration and ends with a transition summary provided to the patient's PCP, including progress toward goals and identification of unresolved issues.[11] Let's see how a patient would be transitioned using this model.

Mrs. M is a 66-year-old patient admitted to the hospital with hyperglycemia. She begins working with Cindy, a clinical nurse specialist certified in gerontology. Cindy conducts some baseline assessments and reviews Mrs. M's chart. Mrs. M's glucose level is greater than 400, and her A1C is 13.8. She has several comorbidities, including hyperlipidemia, diabetes, hypertension, cardiomyopathy, and chronic back pain. She is often distressed by constipation, probably related to her regular use of opiates for back pain. Her Mini-Mental State Exam (MMSE) score is 27/30; Lawton Instrumental Activities of Daily Living (IADL) score is 5/8; KATZ Activities of Daily Living (ADL) is 4/5; and her Geriatric Depression Scale (GDS) score is 1/15.

Therefore, Mrs. M seems to be cognitively intact but is having difficulty with some independent living activities. She walks with a cane and is not depressed. The Patient Activation Measure (PAM) places her at level 2; she is building knowledge and confidence. The literacy screen indicates Mrs. M may have difficulty with basic computation necessary for monitoring her diet and adjusting her medications. She has a limited budget and tells her transitional care nurse, Cindy, that she can't afford her medications. In fact, Mrs. M discloses that she doesn't take any of her medications regularly because of her financial issues. She hit the Medicare "donut hole" last year. Cindy capitalizes on the availability of several members of the clinical care team in the hospital and asks for their recommendations regarding Mrs. M's diabetes control, back pain, and her inability to pay for medications. She also makes sure the discharge planner is aware of Mrs. M's functional limitations.

The clinical dietician makes recommendations to Mrs. M regarding diet for weight, glucose control, and relief of constipation. In addition, she instructs Mrs. M on appropriate portion sizes and reading nutrition labels. Given Mrs. M's difficulty with numeracy, Cindy plans to augment this teaching throughout the intervention. The physical therapist makes recommendations to the bedside nursing staff regarding frequent repositioning and ambulation to maintain physical function and help manage the back pain and constipation. Cindy asks the clinical pharmacist for recommendations regarding whether Mrs. M's drug regimen can be adjusted to be more cost-effective. The clinical pharmacist makes several recommendations that can be discussed with Mrs. M's PCP.

Moreover, the clinical pharmacist recommends some methods for purchasing medications that will assist Mrs. M in reducing her cost. In the meantime, Cindy asks the hospitalist to be mindful of Mrs. M's financial constraints when ordering new medications on discharge.

The day after discharge, Cindy visits Mrs. M at home. Her primary goal is to ensure Mrs. M understands and is following the discharge instructions. Cindy also verifies that Mrs. M has obtained her discharge medications, and they reconcile medications by completing a medication list. Finally, Cindy makes sure Mrs. M has appointments with her PCP and the outpatient diabetes clinic.

In preparation for the first post-discharge appointment with the PCP, Cindy calls to review what Mrs. M would like to achieve during the visit and encourages her to take an active role. Cindy also reminds Mrs. M to bring all of her medications to the appointment. During the office visit, Cindy listens carefully so she can reinforce the physician's instructions during transition visits. After Mrs. M expresses concern regarding her ability to pay for all of her medications, the physician adjusts the medication regimen as necessary, referring to the clinical pharmacist's recommendations.

During additional home and phone visits, Cindy reinforces the diabetic teaching conducted at the outpatient diabetes clinic, encourages ambulation, emphasizes maintaining the medication regimen, and continues to discuss navigating the healthcare system. Because of the volume of issues Mrs. M is trying to manage, as well as her literacy level, Cindy structures the intervention into small components to prevent overwhelming Mrs. M.

Ten weeks later, Mrs. M's glucose levels have improved, her dependence on pain medication is reduced, and she is walking in the shopping mall for exercise. Mrs. M tells Cindy that she feels much better. Cindy will reassess and discharge Mrs. M and send a summary note to Mrs. M's PCP.

Mrs. M—Transitional Care Strategies

- Facilitate Mrs. M's new knowledge in small, frequent components to make it easier for her to assimilate.

- Support and encourage her efforts to take charge of her health.

- Use the expertise of the team to provide Mrs. M with the best input.

- Focus the intervention on those issues most likely to lead to functional decline and rehospitalization.

Expected outcomes

As Dr. Coleman mentioned in the introduction, there are few measures of quality related to transitions. Outcome data can be difficult for decision-makers at a single institution to collect and analyze because some of the most meaningful outcomes occur once a patient has left the purview of the institution. However, there is some meaningful research that has been conducted on transitions programming that should receive serious consideration by decision-makers. In addition, depending on the priorities of the organization, there are other data that could be analyzed.

Readmissions

The most fundamental outcome associated with transitions programs is a reduction in hospitalizations. A randomized controlled trial conducted by Coleman and colleagues found that patients who participated in the Care Transitions Intervention[SM] had lower hospitalization rates at 30, 90, and 180 days after an initial discharge. Further, hospital costs for patients who were admitted to the hospital at 180 days were lower than for controls.[12] Let's check in with our first patient, Mr. D, at 180 days post-discharge.

Approximately 180 days after Mr. D's initial discharge from the hospital, Diane receives a report that he has been admitted. After checking in on Mr. D and reviewing his case with the cardiologist, Diane learns that Mr. D has been admitted with an exacerbation of his congestive heart failure. However, his cardiologist feels Mr. D is in much better shape than he generally is during hospitalizations and that he seems to be using much more effective self-management strategies. In fact, this is the greatest time between hospitalizations since his initial diagnosis. Mr. D tells Diane that he feels much more confident about his ability to assess how he is feeling and when to access care. When Diane reviews the case after discharge, she finds that Mr. D's length of stay is one day shorter than in previous admissions. His cost of care is lower as a result of the shorter length of stay and reduced number of tests during the hospitalization. She reflects that this is probably because his condition was being managed better and the clinical team could feel more confident that Mr. D was following their discharge instructions much more effectively.

A randomized clinical trial conducted by Naylor and associates evaluated the effectiveness of the Transitional Care Program and found intervention participants were less likely to be readmitted, remained out of the hospital for longer periods of time and experienced fewer hospital days. Further, Medicare reimbursements were 50% lower for intervention participants.[13]

The Care Transitions Measure (CTM™)

The Care Transitions Measure (CTM™) is a patient-centered survey instrument designed to assess the quality of care transitions across healthcare settings. It was developed with input from consumers and is self-reported.[14] The CTM elicits patients' feedback regarding their perceived level of involvement in the care process and readiness for self-management. Low CTM scores have been shown to be a predictor of recidivism, both to the hospital and the emergency department. Therefore, some clinicians use the CTM to assess risk of rehospitalization on discharge. It can also be used to measure the effectiveness of efforts to ready patients for self-management. The CTM has been endorsed by the National Quality Forum.[15]

Patient satisfaction

Another possible outcome of the Care Transitions Intervention is an increased rate of patient satisfaction. At my facility, we have received high rates of patient satisfaction scoring since implementing this program. Anecdotally, patients request their transition nurse when they visit the hospital for any reason, even those visits unrelated to their chronic illness. Patients liken it to having a daughter who is a nurse that they can ask to translate the difficult medical information or help navigate a complex healthcare process.

Physician engagement

Physicians often request or write an order for transition nurse services at my hospital. In addition, I have heard physicians tell their patients, "You are really lucky to have a transition coach."

Quality improvement

Medication discrepancies are a key issue addressed in the Care Transition Intervention. If discrepancies are tracked and grouped in a systematic fashion, quality improvement efforts can address the high-volume or high-risk issues. I have experienced a statistically significant decline in medication discrepancies tracked through my transition program by addressing them through quality improvement processes.

Other outcomes tracked could include volume of acute care visits, functional status, laboratory values, achievement of patient goals, and costs. A determination should be made regarding the relative importance of various outcomes to the implementation team and leaders who will approve funding of the program.

Practical Considerations

There are some key factors to think about and plan for when implementing a transition program. Beginning strategically, it is important to determine what your organization hopes to accomplish by implementing a transition program. This can help you measure success and justify future efforts. Suggestions have been provided for outcome indicators. However, a great deal of consideration must be given to the organization's priorities. Most organizational decision-makers will be interested in how a new program affects clinical, service, and financial outcomes. It is important to know how your key decision-makers will judge the program's success.

Healthcare organizations will invest in a transitions program for a variety of reasons. In a managed care market, the financial impact of reducing hospital utilization is obvious. However, there are benefits even in a fee-for-service market. Reducing emergency department overcrowding and making room for more profitable patients could justify a transition program in a hospital with high volumes. Reimbursement and the regulatory environment are providing increasing incentives for smooth handoffs, better communication among providers, and programming to improve patient self-management. Softer, but no less important, are the contributions these programs make to enhancing an organization's community image. Transitions programs can improve patient loyalty and relationships with other providers.

You can make the cost-benefit argument for both approaches. A transition coach is a relatively inexpensive intervention. Costs to consider include salary, laptop, cell phone, travel reimbursement, and patient materials.

A transitional care nurse is more expensive since you will need to pay for the advanced practice expertise and the intervention is longer. A transitional care nurse may need to handle a smaller caseload and will incur additional travel costs.

You may want to establish an oversight team to provide guidance regarding the direction of the program and advocate for the program with key constituents. Think about involving key leaders who may ultimately decide to continue funding of the program. Because the transition nurse needs to be an integral part of the clinical team, you may want to involve some frontline physicians, nurses, and allied healthcare professionals as well. Consider staff who tend to embrace new concepts and can think outside organizational silos when developing new programs. These are the people who will likely provide valuable input and will support the effort overall.

A typical transition coach can handle 24 to 28 patients at a time. As mentioned, the transitional care nurse may have a smaller caseload. Generally, the caseload is composed of patients in three phases: 1/3 currently in the hospital, 1/3 in the home visit phase, and 1/3 receiving follow-up phone calls. This is true for both programs. Therefore, if you are able to begin with just one coach, you may want to consider beginning on one clinical service. This will provide you with enough volume in a specific patient population to exhibit meaningful outcomes. If you decide to begin this way, select a clinical service with a strong leader and interested physicians. It will set you up for success if you can ally yourself with a strong team.

Perhaps the most important consideration is who to hire as the transition coach or nurse. Functioning in this role requires that the clinician is an excellent communicator and a true believer in patient self-management. If implementing the Transitional Care Model, the nurse must also have excellent clinical skills in order to assess patient needs, recommend improvements, provide clinical information, and implement evidence-based protocols. It is also important to hire someone who is comfortable working independently within the healthcare system. Someone who has experience in hospital and home settings will have a shorter learning curve than someone who has worked in just one care environment. Also, keep in mind that the transition nurse or coach will need to manage multiple patients with diverse needs who are at different points in the process. However, the most important consideration is to hire someone who can facilitate and coach, rather than do. The goal of both of these programs is to support patient self-management. Patient self-management is unlikely to occur if the transition coach is continuing to do everything for the patient. This cannot be overemphasized. It is often the hardest thing for anyone new to the role.

A Final Word

Both Dr. Coleman and Dr. Naylor offer highly useful information on their websites. They include components of the programs, tools, and information that are helpful in building the business case. Access *caretransitions.org* for the Care Transitions Intervention and *transitionalcare.info* for the Transitional Care model. In addition, Drs. Coleman and Naylor offer excellent training programs for staff interested in the roles of transition coach or transitional care nurse. Visit their websites for more information.

References

1. E.A. Coleman, J.D. Smith, J.C. Frank, S.J. Min, C. Parry, A.M. Kramer, "Preparing Patients and Caregivers to Participate in Care Delivered Across Settings: The Care Transitions Intervention," *Journal of American Geriatrics Society* 52 (2004): 1817–1825.

2. C. Parry, E.A. Coleman, J. Smith, J. Frank, A. Kramer, A "The Care Transitions Intervention: A Patient-Centered Approach to Ensuring Effective Transfers Between Sites of Geriatric Care," *Home Health Services Quarterly*, 22 (2003): 1–17.

3. National Council on Patient Information and Education, *Enhancing Prescription Medicine Adherence: A National Action Plan, August 2007* (Rockville, MD: NCPIE, 2007).

4. C. Parry, E.A. Coleman, J. Smith, J. Frank, A. Kramer, A "The Care Transitions Intervention: A Patient-Centered Approach to Ensuring Effective Transfers Between Sites of Geriatric Care," *Home Health Services Quarterly*, 22 (2003): 1–17.

5. See note 1 above.

6. S.F. Jencks, M.V. Williams, E.A. Coleman, "Rehospitalizations Among Patients in the Medicare Fee-for-Service Program," *New England Journal of Medicine*, 360 (2009): 1418–28.

7. See note 2 above.

8. Institute of Medicine, *Leading Health Indicators for Healthy People 2010: Final Report (1999) Institute of Medicine (IOM) Leading Health Indicators for Healthy People 2010: Final Report* Released: April 7, 2003 Type: Consensus Report, (Washington, DC: The National Academies Press)

9. C. Parry, E.A. Coleman, J. Smith, J. Frank, A. Kramer, A "The Care Transitions Intervention: A Patient-Centered Approach to Ensuring Effective Transfers Between Sites of Geriatric Care," *Home Health Services Quarterly*, 22 (2003): 1–17.

10. M.D. Naylor, D. Brooten, R. Campbell, B.S. Jacobsen, M.D. Mezey, M.V. Pauley, et al., "Comprehensive Discharge Planning and Home Follow-Up of Hospitalized Elders: A Randomized Clinical Trial," *JAMA*, 281 (1999): 613–620.

11. Transitional Care Model. *http://transitionalcare.info/* accessed April 1, 2010.

12. E.A. Coleman, C. Parry, S. Chalmers, S.J. Min, "The Care Transitions Intervention: Results of a Randomized Controlled Trial," Archives of Internal Medicine, 166 (2006): 1822–1828.

13. See note 10 above.

14. E.A. Coleman, J.D. Smith, J.C. Frank, T.B. Eilertsen, J.N. Thiare, A.M. Kramer, "Development and Testing of a Measure Designed to Assess the Quality of Care Transitions," *International Journal of Integrated Care* Vol. 2, 1 June 2002.

15. E.A. Coleman, C. Parry C, S. Chalmers, A. Chugh, E. Mahoney, "The Central Role of Performance Measurement in Improving the Quality of Transitional Care," *Home Healthcare Service Quarterly*, 26 (2007): 93–104.

Caregivers: Holding Transitions Together

LEARNING OBJECTIVES

After reading this chapter, you should be able to:

- Discuss the value of caregiving to society and the personal cost to the caregiver

- Evaluate caregiver assessments and incorporate one into your practice

- Describe the elements of an educational process for caregivers

For children, caregivers are treated as an integral part of the clinical care process. In the healthcare system for adults, however, family and friends who give of themselves as caregivers are the unsung heroes. Too often, they play an unrecognized, solitary role in managing the complex process of transitions. Caregivers can be the only ones coordinating the process of accessing care from a multitude of providers and ensuring needed treatments. They are also a critical information conduit among providers who do not communicate with one another. In addition, caregivers are sometimes the only ones who recognize when care plans conflict.[1] The clinical care process demands even more from caregivers as aging patients are discharged from hospitals with chronic care needs.

The Value of Caregiving

The average caregiver provides the equivalent of a half-time workweek in assistance.[2] The 2008 Update from AARP's Public Policy Institute valued this unpaid work at $375 billion in 2007. Just how much is $375 billion a year? To put it in perspective, $375 billion is more than total Medicare spending over the same period, more than the total 2007 sales of Wal-Mart, and more than $1,000 for every person in the United States.[3] Caregiving is a valuable commodity.

The cost of caregiving, however, is personal. Sometimes caregivers have to stop working for pay. Midlife women in the labor force often leave because of caregiving responsibilities.[4] In fact, 37% of caregivers of people over the age of 50 either leave the workforce or find it necessary to reduce their hours.[5] Stress, too, takes its toll. We now have decades of evidence of the physical and mental effects of caregiving. Clearly, stress tends to increase as the demands of caring for an aging population increase.[6] In addition, caregivers spend more than their time. Caregivers of people over age 50 reportedly spent an average of $5,531 out of pocket in 2007.[7]

The benefit of caregiving to the healthcare system is significant and can be translated into dollars. People who have caregivers tend to have shorter hospital stays.[8] Patients without caregivers are more likely to be readmitted.[9] The presence of a caregiver tends to reduce nursing home use.[10]

It simply does not make sense for the healthcare system to continue to ignore this crucial part of the patient care team. The Institute of Medicine, in its 2007 report, *Retooling for an Aging America: Building the Healthcare Workforce*, asserts that older adults must be recognized as active participants in the healthcare process.[11] For those adults who cannot be active participants, caregivers must be accepted as an integral part of the team.

Investing in Caregivers

In order for patients and caregivers to participate actively in the transition process, an investment should be made in their knowledge base. Education related to the tasks they are required to perform could increase confidence and decrease stress. Caregivers often leave the hospital panicked by the complex responsibilities they are ill-prepared to assume, yet many are afraid to admit their limitations. Therefore, the first step for healthcare professionals should be to assess the abilities of the caregiver.

The Caregiver Assessment: General Guidelines

Who is the caregiver?

It is sometimes difficult to determine who the caregiver of an older adult is; therefore, the first step is to identify the caregiver. Often, simply asking, "Who is your caregiver?" does not produce a satisfactory response, particularly in the event that the older adult has several children, a spouse, and perhaps additional relatives and friends. It is more effective to ask specific questions related to the care a patient is likely to need. Questions may include:

- Who picks up your medicines? Assists you in taking them?

- Who helps with your medical equipment?

- Who helps you do the grocery shopping? Prepare meals?

- Who goes to the doctor with you?

If several people assist, a determination of how frequently specific caregivers are involved may be necessary. And, of course, it is important to ask the patient about his or her preferences.[12, 13]

The assessment domains

Once the caregiver, or caregivers, are identified, the assessment of his current role, strengths, and need for enrichment can begin. According to the National Center on Caregiving at Family Caregiver Alliance (FCA), a caregiving assessment is

> *A systematic process of gathering information that describes a caregiving situation and identifies the particular problems, needs, resources and strengths of the family caregiver. It approaches issues from the caregiver's perspective and culture, focuses on what assistance the caregiver may need and the outcomes the family member wants for support, and seeks to maintain the caregiver's own health and well-being.*[14]

This definition emphasizes the caregiver as a central part of the healthcare team, along with the patient. Also, it pushes the medical community to systematically analyze the caregiving relationship. We can no longer assume orders can be carried out just as they are written in a discharge plan. There needs to be an interchange of information between the medical team and the caregiver-patient team.

The FCA national consensus conference outlined several domains to include in a caregiver assessment. The Next Step in Care program of the United Hospital Fund reflects these in the guidance it provides on caregiver assessment. Both resources will be used in this section. The broad domains included in a caregiver assessment include context, caregiver's perception of health and functional status of care recipient, caregiver values and preferences, well-being of the caregiver, consequences of caregiving, skills/abilities/knowledge to provide care recipient with needed care, and potential resources that caregivers may choose to use (**Figure 6.1**).

Figure 6.1

Domains of the Caregiver Assessment

Define the context of the patient-caregiver relationship.
Identify the caregiver's perception of the health and functional status of the patient.
Discover the caregiver's values and preferences.
Evaluate the wellbeing of the caregiver.
Identify the consequences of caregiving for this particular caregiver.
Assess the caregiver's knowledge, skills and abilities.
Identify potential resources the caregiver could use.

Context

The first step in assessing the caregiver is to define the context of the patient-caregiver relationship. Elements include the relationship of the caregiver to the patient and the quality of the family relationships. It is helpful to ascertain how long the caregiver has been caring for the patient and whether the caregiver works outside the caregiving relationship. Practical information related to the physical environment; the number of people in the home; and the financial status, age, and education of the caregiver are also important contextual considerations. After obtaining basic information, it may be important to ask the caregiver the following questions:

- How many stairs are there into your home? Is the patient's bedroom on an upper floor?

- Do you have a shower or bathtub?

- What are the ages of the people who live in your home?

- Do you work outside of the home? Volunteer?

- What level of education did you complete?

- Do you have caregiving responsibilities for anyone else? Does the patient?

Caregiver's perception of health and functional status of health recipient

Early in the assessment, it is important to determine the caregiver's perception of the health and functional status of the patient. Include questions about the patient's abilities related to activities of daily living and instrumental activities of daily living. Also, inquire about the patient's level of need related to medical tests and procedures. It is also important to assess the caregiver's view of the patient's psychosocial needs, cognition, and behavioral issues. Consider asking the caregiver the following questions:

- How much assistance do you give the patient while toileting, ambulating, and bathing?

- How much assistance do you give the patient with paying bills, and managing her checking account?

- How does the patient view his level of independence?

Caregiver values and preferences

Do not make assumptions about the caregiver's willingness to provide care or assume that he or she has unlimited availability for medical appointments. Assess the degree of interest and perceptions of the obligation, as well as preferences for hospital aftercare. Determine the patient's willingness to accept assistance. Also, remember to ask about related cultural considerations. Consider asking the following questions:

+ How often do you assist the patient in getting to medical appointments? Are you comfortable with that?

+ Are you able to accompany the patient to the follow-up appointment with Dr. Jones on February 4 at 2:00 p.m.?

+ Are there special religious or cultural considerations we should take into consideration for your family?[15, 16]

Well-being of the caregiver

According to the American Association for Marriage and Family Therapy, 80% of caregivers say they feel a great deal of stress and 50% are clinically depressed. It is important not to overlook the health and well-being of the caregiver. Allow the caregiver to provide a self-rating of his or her health and evaluate its impact on the caregiving process. Include any health conditions, emotional issues (including depression and anxiety), and perceived quality of life.[17]

The Hartford Institute of Geriatric Nursing has a wonderful online series of assessments, including their evidence base, and a description of how to use them. The website contains the Modified Caregiver Strain Index (CSI) that would provide valuable information related to this section of the caregiver assessment. The CSI is a 13-item questionnaire used to quickly screen for caregiver strain and its sources. It can be used with caregivers of any age and was tested with a sample of 158 family caregivers providing assistance to adults age 53 and older living in a community-based setting. The domains include Employment, Financial, Physical, Social, and Time.

The strengths of the instrument include its ease of use and straightforward language. Further, caregivers are permitted to rank each domain according to "Yes—on a regular basis," "Yes—sometimes," and "No," allowing for a middle ground that may more accurately reflect reality or may be a more comfortable answer. The instrument is limited in that there is no definition of a low, medium, or high stratum of strain. The professional judgment of the screener will guide his determination of the next steps.

However, the CSI does identify those caregivers in need of support. High scores indicate that further probing should occur and support should be provided. Specific areas of concern would be indicated by the domains rated "Yes" by the caregiver.[18]

Consequences of caregiving

In order to assess the consequences of caregiving, ask the caregiver about his perceptions of the challenges and benefits associated with caregiving. Some of the perceived challenges would have been identified with the Modified Caregiver Strain Index. Additional probing questions could include the following:

- How does taking care of your mother affect your daily life?

- What do you enjoy doing in your spare time? Are you able to do the things you enjoy and take care of your father?

Knowledge needed to provide care recipient with needed care

Evaluate the skill of the caregiver by asking specific questions about the ability to successfully carry out necessary tasks related to the medical needs of the patient. This should also determine the degree of confidence felt by the caregiver. Consider asking specific questions related to the tasks the caregiver will need to perform at home:

- Has anyone shown you how to assist your mother in getting from her bed to the walker without injuring yourself?

- Has anyone shown you and your mother how to correctly use the walker?

- Do you feel comfortable doing these things?

Additional questions can follow this same general pattern. If possible, it is ideal to watch the caregiver perform these tasks before discharge in order to provide direct coaching before the tasks need to be performed outside your watchful eye.

Potential resources for the caregiver

Finally, ask about the caregiver's knowledge regarding resources available for assistance. Ask specific questions related to resources that might be helpful given the needs of the patient and caregiver:

+ Are you familiar with the Alzheimer's Association? They would be very helpful to you and your uncle. Would you be interested in learning more about our local chapter?

+ Are you familiar with the AARP website? The AARP has resources on family caregiving and an online discussion group that you may find helpful. Would you like the Internet address?[19, 20]

The United Hospital Fund's Next Step in Care program has an online assessment self-assessment tool for family caregivers. It covers each of the caregiver assessment domains and asks specific questions in lay terms. Caregivers are asked to identify what activities of daily living and instrumental activities of daily living need to be performed for their loved one. Caregivers also identify which tasks they need training to be able to perform and which tasks they are unable to perform.

The assessment then asks the caregiver to identify services his or her loved one had before this hospital admission. It may be necessary to explain any new services that are called for so the caregiver knows how and when to access them. This may also encourage the caregiver to ask about services that have not been recommended but are needed.

There is a section entitled "About Worries," which can be used to begin a discussion about caregiver strain. It is an unobtrusive assessment that will likely prompt discussion without making the caregiver feel guilty. The next section asks the caregiver to identify resources and people who are available for help. This should encourage caregivers to think about their well-being and help them realize that it is okay to ask for assistance.

The assessment can be saved to a local hard drive or printed.[21]

A Homecare Assessment Tool

The Visiting Nurse Service of New York has developed a caregiver assessment that can be used in the transition from the hospital to homecare. The "Let's PREPARE" instrument has been made available online through the Hartford Institute for Geriatric Nursing.

Psychometric testing has not been done; however, the "Let's PREPARE" instrument was developed by a panel of expert homecare nurses and addresses many issues that must be faced by informal caregivers. It includes the areas often covered by home care nurses on their first visit. The target population is informal caregivers of older adults receiving homecare.

The categories included in the "Let's PREPARE" instrument are:

- Prescriptions

    - Is there a plan for obtaining and paying for needed medications?

    - Is the caregiver knowledgeable about the medications?

    - Is the caregiver able to administer the medications?

- Readiness to manage at home

    - Is the caregiver knowledgeable and prepared with regard to the hospital discharge plan and any orders for follow-up, including primary care appointments, medical testing, necessary insurance, supplies and equipment necessary, etc.?

    - Are any modifications to the home necessary to prevent injury to the patient or allow for medical treatments?

    - Does the caregiver have contact information for the medical team providing ongoing care and other community resources?

- Early changes in condition

  - Is the caregiver knowledgeable about the patient's medical issues, warning signs of a deteriorating condition, and when to access care?

- Partnership among the home health team

  - Does the caregiver know who will be providing professional care at home and who to access for specific needs?

- Assistance needed to perform procedures

  - What assistance does the caregiver need to perform necessary medical or daily living tasks for the patient?

- Realistic expectations and goals

  - Does the caregiver have any psychosocial, behavioral, or medical issues that might interfere with providing the care needed at home?

- Education and empowerment

  - What topics does the caregiver need to be educated on to fulfill the role with confidence?

  - Does the caregiver have a contingency plan if needed services do not arrive on time?

General information within the categories has been provided. If interested in incorporating this process into your practice, access the complete instrument online.[22]

The Assessment Process

Some caregivers feel put off by an assessment and feel it is a challenge to their competency; therefore, it is important to be open and honest about the assessment. It may help to frame the assessment as an interview to help ascertain how the medical team can help with the transition to the next level of care.

The assessment should be conducted as early as possible so the information can be used to plan for transitional care. Further, it may be tempting to assume a constant level of caregiver willingness and ability for patients who are frequent visitors to the hospital. But, situations and medical needs change; thus, a caregiver assessment should be conducted at each hospitalization.

Many healthcare professionals are qualified to conduct a caregiver assessment. More important than the clinical function is the focus on the caregiver as an important partner on the healthcare team. And there are general knowledge, skills, and abilities that are essential. The assessor should possess knowledge regarding the purpose of the assessment, family systems and conflict resolution, resource availability and building of a community support network, aging, self-determination versus safety issues, and the importance of caregiver participation. Skills should include communicating effectively, interviewing, engaging with people (even those who may not want help) and disseminating information clearly. Abilities include listening, handling emotional content, being sensitive to differences, having empathy, being comfortable with a self-management approach, keeping opinions in check, and possessing an understanding that the assessor may not know everything (**Figure 6.2**).[23, 24]

Figure 6.2		

Qualifications to Conduct Assessment

Knowledge	The purpose of the assessment
	Family systems and conflict resolution
	Resource availability and building a community support network
	Aging
	Self determination versus safety issues
	Importance of caregiver participation
Skills	Communicating effectively
	Interviewing
	Engaging with people
	Disseminating information clearly
	Listening
	Handling emotional content
	Sensitivity to differences
Abilities	Empathy
	Comfort with a self management approach
	Keeping opinions in check
	An understanding of not be omniscient

Educating the Caregiver

Once you know what the caregiver's capabilities and needs are, you can provide education related to the role he will be expected to perform. Often, caregivers educate themselves, and many of the resources available are developed for self-directed learners. Tools intended as self-directed learning for caregivers can be useful as a framework for professionals interested in creating an educational program. At a minimum, these tools should be provided to caregivers in preparation for the transition process.

As you are educating caregivers, it is important to remember the adult learning principles.

- **The need to know.** Be sure the caregiver knows your intent is to help him with information that will be useful as soon as he gets home with his loved one. Whet the caregiver's appetite by providing a suggestion related to something he may be worried about or struggling with based upon the caregiver assessment.

- **The learner's self-concept.** Make the caregiver an active participant in the process. Ask questions. Ask him to show you something or repeat what he understands about what you have said.

- **The role of the learner's experience.** Engage the caregiver in the process by asking about how he and the patient manage specific tasks now. Ask in a way that conveys your interest in his (or the patient's) preferences, not in a way that makes him think you are challenging his caregiving competence.

- **Readiness to learn.** Remember, people will be ready to learn things that will help them now, not at some point in the future. Don't overwhelm the caregiver by teaching him all the things he will need to know for the next 20 years of caring for his loved one. Emphasize the things the caregiver will need to know immediately upon discharge and make sure the caregiver knows who he can access for additional questions once they get home.

- **Orientation to learning.** Make the educational experience as meaningful as possible. When you can, teach the caregiver at the bedside using equipment and supplies they will use at home.

- **Motivation.** Remember to meet the caregiver where they are. The caregiver assessment should give you some idea of how the caregiver views his role. Work with what you have, not with your view of the ideal caregiver.[25]

After-hospital appointments and services

The Centers for Medicare and Medicaid Services (CMS) has a checklist for discharge that provides a useful framework for caregiver education in preparation for a hospital discharge to home. Visit *Medicare.gov* and download *Planning for Your Discharge* from the landing page. To illustrate caregiver education, we'll follow Mrs. G, her nurse, Stephanie, and her caregiver, Shirley, as they prepare for discharge. We'll use the CMS checklist and the adult education principles as resources to guide us.

Caregivers must know what the expectations are for care after discharge and who will be providing services. This is an area that can be overwhelming. Generally, older adults have several post-discharge appointments and may have testing or treatments that must be performed after discharge. Let's get to know Mrs. G's team and see how they handle this.

Mrs. G is an 87-year-old woman who was hospitalized after suffering a stroke. This has left her with weakness on her left side and difficulty ambulating. In addition, she is now on anticoagulation therapy. Mrs. G lives with her daughter, Shirley, a 66-year-old widow and retired physical education teacher. Mrs. G's nurse, Stephanie, is preparing mother and daughter for discharge home. Stephanie has performed a caregiver assessment and brings that to the meeting in Mrs. G's room.

Stephanie knows that the neurologist caring for Mrs. G in the hospital wants to see her in the office a few days after discharge and will follow her care on an ongoing basis. He orders homecare for nursing and physical therapy services. He also orders Mrs. G to begin using a walker. Stephanie makes sure Mrs. G and Shirley have the date, time, and location of the first post-discharge appointment. Stephanie verifies that this works with Shirley's schedule and they have transportation to the appointment. Stephanie then ensures Mrs. G and Shirley know who will be visiting from homecare and the durable medical equipment provider, as well as what each agency will be doing. Stephanie makes sure Shirley has contact numbers, just in case the providers don't come when she expects them or arrangements need to change.

Beginning this way satisfies Shirley's need to know something she is ready to learn because it will happen soon after discharge. It is also a fairly low-risk discussion to have and can establish Stephanie as a person with information who wants to help.

Mrs. G—Caregiver Education Strategies

- **Need to know:** Begin by providing education related to something Shirley is worried about. Meet her most pressing needs first.

- **Role of the learner's experience:** Use Shirley's knowledge of body mechanics and experience in caring for her mother as a foundation from which to build in the teaching process.

- **Readiness to learn:** Shirley will need to attend to activities of daily living immediately upon arriving home so make sure she is comfortable with those tasks.

- **Orientation to learning:** Use the materials Shirley will need to use at home when you are educating her in the hospital.

- **Learner's self concept:** Make Shirley an active participant. Have her try some of the tasks under your watchful eye.

- **Motivation:** Shirley seems motivated to learn to care for her mother upon discharge from this hospitalization. Remember to check this during each hospitalization and encourage Shirley to find a way to take some time off.

Aftercare equipment and daily living assistance

While they are on the subject of durable medical equipment, the nurse could take the opportunity to make sure the caregiver knows how to use the equipment he will need at home. This may also be an ideal time to check about assistance with activities of daily living and instrumental activities of daily living.

Stephanie takes the walker at Mrs. G's bedside and asks Shirley if anyone has instructed her how to use it. Shirley seems uncertain, so Stephanie provides a concise explanation of the purpose of a walker and how it works. Stephanie then demonstrates how to assist Mrs. G in getting out of bed to the walker and how to assist with ambulation. Stephanie watches as Shirley tries these tasks and provides guidance through the process. Because Shirley is a retired physical education teacher, she has a strong foundation for body mechanics and asks good questions. Stephanie makes use of this knowledge and builds upon it as it relates to Mrs. G and her equipment.

Shirley seems motivated to assist her mother and learn as much as she can, so Stephanie can make good use of this in the teaching relative to the walker and other topics. Stephanie has also used Shirley's experience as a retired physical education teacher and has engaged her in the learning by using equipment that will be needed at home and allowing Shirley to practice. Stephanie then transitions to a discussion about assisting Mrs. G with other activities like bathing, dressing, and toileting. Mrs. G handled many of her own instrumental activities of daily living before the hospitalization, so Stephanie discusses changes in cognition that may occur following a stroke and recommends a follow-up discussion with the neurologist. Stephanie doesn't want to overwhelm Shirley by discussing things that may never happen. She remembers people are ready to learn things they will need to know right away.

The diagnosis

The nurse should also review the new diagnosis with the caregiver to make sure he or she knows what to expect and how to identify signs of a deteriorating condition. Caregivers should know what the warning signs are and how to access care should they occur.

Stephanie continues the discussion by providing a brief explanation of what happens during an ischemic stroke, which Mrs. G experienced. Stephanie uses a color illustration of the brain to assist in the explanation. She includes a description of some of the physical and cognitive effects of a stroke and makes sure Shirley knows what to watch out for. She then asks Shirley to explain the warning signs in her own words. Stephanie also asks Shirley to identify which members of the medical team she would access for various warning signs.

In using the illustration of the brain and asking Shirley related questions, Stephanie has created an orientation to learning that engaged Shirley in the process and made it as meaningful as possible.

Medications

This can be the most complex area for caregivers. Older adults are often on a plethora of medications, prescribed by different providers and administered according to a variety of instructions. Caregivers need to be knowledgeable about the administration and purpose of the medications, as well as what the potential side effects are. Since they also need to obtain and pay for the medications, the treatment team needs to make sure caregivers can manage all of this.

Stephanie now moves onto the medications Mrs. G will need to take after discharge. She asks Shirley to identify the medications Mrs. G was taking before her admission and how she was taking them. Stephanie also asks about obtaining and paying for the medications. In this way, Stephanie has made use of Shirley's experience and has identified the areas she does not need to review.

Mrs. G. will be started on oral anticoagulation therapy at home. Stephanie makes sure Shirley knows how to administer the warfarin and what to watch out for. She also makes sure Shirley knows how important it is to take Mrs. G to have her PT/INR monitored. And, Stephanie reviews drug interactions and diet with Shirley. In order to check for understanding, Stephanie asks Shirley specific questions about transportation for the monitoring and how she will handle Mrs. G's diet. Stephanie has made Shirley an active participant in the learning process.

Caregiver well-being

As previously mentioned, caregivers cannot do their job without taking care of themselves. The professional staff should not overlook the opportunity to explore how the caregiver is coping and how she views her situation.

Stephanie asks Shirley about how she feels about the new tasks she will be required to perform and whether she has a plan for backup and respite. Shirley has adult children who live nearby but she has been hesitant about asking them to help with the care for Mrs. G. Stephanie encourages Shirley to ask so that she can get out on the golf course from time to time to rejuvenate herself.[26, 27]

What Happens When the Caregiver and the Patient Don't Agree?

The assumption so far has been that caregiver and patient have the same goals and agree on the decisions that affect the caregiving relationship. The reality is, this isn't always the case. Disagreements between caregivers and their loved ones is a tough issue, and there are few resources for guidance. Perhaps because this is a more common concern in patients with dementia, the FCA provides suggestions related to this population. These suggestions can serve as general guidance.

Research shows the caregiving relationship is most satisfying when the care provided closely matches the patient's values and preferences. Caregivers want to do what their loved ones want. This can often form the foundation for a healing discussion. A trained professional, such as a social worker or family therapist, should facilitate discussions like these.

The therapist will likely begin with an assessment that focuses on the care preferences and values of each participant and then work with the participant to foster mutual understanding. The discussion will include preferences for details related to daily life, such as living and financial arrangements. Both parties will be encouraged to participate in the assessment and the care plan.

The therapist will recognize the caregiver's need for information, emotional support, and help. The therapist will also keep an open mind about the family relationship and encourage each party to recognize one another's rights to make their own life choices, even when there might be disagreement about those choices.[28]

Coaching the Caregiver Instead of the Patient

The Care Transition Intervention[SM] is useful for the caregiver as well as the patient. When there is a caregiver who will be managing the activities related to the four pillars, the caregiver is coached. The coach can assess the caregiver's level of activation, literacy, current practices, and baseline knowledge. The coach can then progress through the coaching process during the hospitalization, home visits, and follow-up phone calls. If the patient is able to participate, the coach will involve him or her as much as possible.

The Future of Caregiving

The overall availability of family caregivers in the United States is declining. Causes postulated are the overwhelming number of women in the paid workforce, families living farther apart, and the declining population of younger family members. Many caregivers are spouses, who are themselves aging. Forty-seven percent of spousal caregivers are 75 years and older.

As the availability of family caregivers is decreasing, the number of people in need of caregiving is increasing. As the population ages, so does the incidence of chronic disease, which requires ongoing management outside the professional healthcare system. These factors accentuate the need for caregiver support. The strategies discussed here—assessment, education, and emotional support—form the path to a successful patient-professional-caregiver relationship (**Figure 6.3**).[29]

Figure 6.3

The Path to a Successful Caregiving Relationship

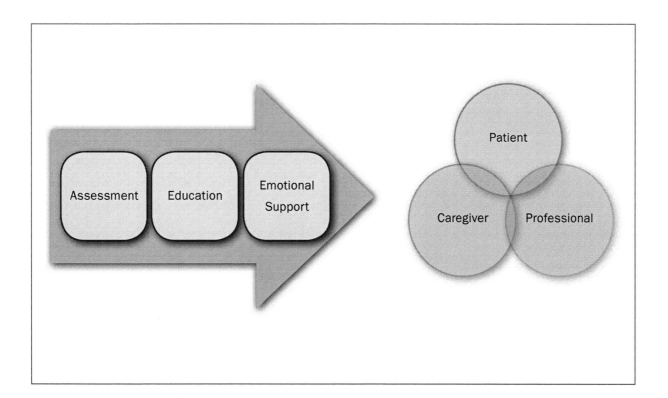

References

1. Institute of Medicine, Retooling for an Aging America, (Washington DC: The National Academies Press, 2008).

2. R.W. Johnson and J.M. Wiener, A Profile of Frail Older Americans and Their Caregivers, The Retirement Project, Occasional Paper No. 8, (Washington, DC: The Urban Institute, 2006).

3. AARP Public Policy Institute. Insight on the Issues. Valuing the Invaluable: the Economic Value of Family Caregiving, 2008 Update. Issue 13, November 2008. Available at *http://assets.aarp.org/rgcenter/il/i13_caregiving.pdf.*

4. E.K. Pavalko and K.A. Henderson, "Combining Care Work and Paid Work: Do Workplace Policies Make a Difference?" Research on Aging, 28(3): 359–374 (May 2006).

5. Evercare in Collaboration with National Alliance for Caregiving, Family Caregivers – What They Spend, What They Sacrifice: The Personal Financial Toll of Caring for a Loved One, (Minnetonka, MN: Evercare & Bethesda, MD: NAC, 2007).

6. See note 1 above.

7. See note 5 above.

8. G. Picone G, R.M. Wilson, S. Chous, "Analysis of Hospital Length of Stay and Discharge Destination Using Hazard Functions with Unmeasured Heterogeneity," *Health Economics* 12 (2003): 1021–1034.

9. E.C. Schwartz, "Identification of Factors Predictive of Hospital Readmissions for Patients with Heart Failure," *Heart & Lung*, 32 (2003): 88–89.

10. C.H. Van Houten and E.C. Norton, "Informal Care and Medicare Expenditures: Testing for Heterogeneous Treatment Effects," Journal of Health Economics, 27 (2008): 134–156.

11. See note 1 above.

12. National Center on Caregiving at Family Caregiver Alliance, "Caregivers Count Too! A Toolkit to Help Practitioners Assess the Needs of Family Caregivers, June 2006.

13. Next Step in Care, "Assessing Family Caregivers: A Guide for Healthcare Providers," United Hospital Fund 2008.

14. See note 12 above.

15. See note 12 above.

16. See note 13 above.

17. American Association for Marriage and Family Therapy. AAMFT Consumer Update Caregiving for the Elderly, *www.aamft.org/families/consumer_updates/caregiving_elderly.asp* accessed April 19, 2010.

18. Hartford Institute for Geriatric Nursing, Consult GeriRN.org, Try This: Best Practices in Nursing Care to Older Adults, *http://consultgerirn.org/uploads/File/trythis/issue14.pdf*, accessed April 19, 2010.

19. See note 12 above.

20. See note 13 above.

21. United Hospital Fund, Next Step in Care, "What Do I Need as a Family Caregiver?" 2008

22. See note 18 above.

23. See note 12 above.

24. See note 13 above.

25. M. Knowles, The Adult Learner: A Neglected Species, (Houston: Gulf Publishing Company, 1984): 52–61.

26. See note 25 above.

27. Centers for Medicare and Medicaid Services. Planning for Your Discharge: A Checklist for Patients and *Caregivers Preparing to Leave a Hospital, Nursing Home or Other Health Care Setting*, 8/2008, Available at *www.medicare.gov/ publications/pubs/pdf/11376.pdf.*

28. Family Caregiver Alliance, *Helping Families Make Everyday Care Choices (for Providers)*, *www.caregiver.org/caregiver/ jsp/content_node.jsp?nodeid=405* accessed April 19, 2010.

29. See note 1 above.

Nursing Home Transitions and Acute Care Transfer

In general, 17.4% of nursing home residents are transitioned to the hospital in a given six-month period. Hospitalizations for this population are costly and expose residents to iatrogenic complications.[1] To address these issues, the aim is not to improve the patient's self-management capability, but to improve the appropriateness of the transfer and the collaboration between the clinical teams on each end.

The Problem With Acute Care Transfers

A review of the literature on nursing home-emergency department transfers, conducted by Terrell and Miller, found collaboration to be nonexistent to minimal. Nursing home, ambulance, and emergency department professionals all reported significant numbers of patients transferred with no written or verbal communication. When written documentation was provided, often it was not presented in a format or at a time that was useful. These observations were true for all types of transfer: nursing home to ambulance, ambulance to emergency department, and back again. Not surprisingly, the professionals across these transfers reported concern that they are working without adequate background and direction, and that they are not respecting the wishes of the patients. Several solutions were proposed, including exchanging oral summaries dictated on cassette tapes, standardizing reporting formats, and expanding the use of information technology.[2]

Davis and colleagues enumerated the types of communication problems between nursing homes and hospitals that are familiar to anyone working in the field. They ranged from the inability to read handwriting to the lack of a contact person to call with questions. Also included were lack of reports and missing information in reports. Differences in workplace culture were associated with communication problems because the transferring professionals did not understand the constraints faced by their colleagues at the other end. For example, hospital staff did not realize late discharges made it very difficult for nursing homes to obtain needed patient equipment and medications.[3]

Coleman and Fox point out that there is often lack of agreement between settings on what constitutes necessary information. Therefore, each institution develops its own unique intake form, which adds to the inefficiency of the transfer process. They recommend nursing homes and hospitals work in partnership to develop solutions related to some broad categories. First, the institutions should work together to define the core information elements that must be exchanged and develop standard operating processes for communication. The operational processes must include mechanisms for ensuring accountability to provide timely and accurate information. Finally, the communication process must be user-friendly to permit exchange and collaboration across settings.[4]

Although an important type of transition, there have not been many evidence-based programs developed to specifically address this issue. Here, we will describe three programs (outlined in **Figure 7.1**) whose evidence base currently is being formed.

Figure 7.1

Elements of the Models

Evercare	Summa's Care Coordination Network	INTERACT
Primary team model	Consistent nursing facility referral process	Clinical tools that: • Identify early changes in clinical status • Comprehensively assess the resident • Document status changes • Communicate more effectively regarding status changes
Increases the availability of NPs	A single post-acute transfer form	
Increases focus on patient monitoring and care	Electronic referral process	
	Collaboration of 30 healthcare organizations	A process for continuous improvement
		Tools for advance care planning

Evercare

Evercare is a care coordination program of UnitedHealthcare that has been implemented for Medicare and Medicaid beneficiaries in 38 states. It also provides support to more than 700,000 family caregivers through employers across the United States. Evercare uses a primary team model in which nurse practitioners augment the medical care provided by physicians on their team. They can address the commonly occurring fluctuations in the health of frail elders that are often the cause of transfers to the acute care setting.[5] Frail elders are usually hospitalized for infections, adverse events such as falls, exacerbations of chronic illnesses, or uncontrolled pain. These events can be distressing to clinical caregivers and families alike.[6] The limited knowledge base of nursing home frontline staff related to acute illness has been identified as an opportunity for improvement related to reduction of acute care transfers.[7] The Evercare model can address this by increasing the availability of nurse practitioners (NP).

The Evercare model was studied as a demonstration project through the Centers for Medicare and Medicaid Services (CMS) in 1995. CMS then contracted with Dr. Robert Kane, Dean of the University of Minnesota School of Public Health to analyze the effectiveness of the model. The findings result from an analysis of utilization data from five Evercare sites over two years, plus case studies, structured interviews, and surveys conducted by Dr. Kane's team of researchers. Outcomes include a reduction in hospitalizations, emergency room visits, and acute episodes in the nursing home. The identification and treatment of acute illnesses in the nursing home resulted in a 45% reduction in hospitalizations with no change in mortality. Patients who were hospitalized experienced a drop in length of stay by one day. Further, by placing an increased focus on patient monitoring and care, the number of acute care episodes in the nursing home decreased. Emergency room visits diminished by 50%. Dr. Kane concluded the NPs may have prevented some hospitalizations but the primary effect was that the patient cases were handled more cost-effectively. In fact, Dr. Kane estimated that each NP saved about $130,000 per year.[8]

The Evercare model has been piloted by nine primary care trusts in England. The target population was elders at high risk of readmission, and the primary outcome measured was hospital readmission. Several articles have been written about the experience and include similar observations. In this pilot, readmission rates did not experience a statistically significant decline. However, the system in which the model was implemented may have influenced the outcomes.[9, 10] Gravelle and colleagues recommend more sweeping system changes to impact readmission rates in England.[11]

A complete review of the literature on this model can instruct those of us attempting to tackle this difficult issue. Although the results varied, healthcare leaders should evaluate their organizations, identify desired outcomes, and then select the approach that seems most beneficial to their unique circumstances.

Summa's Care Coordination Network

An increasing demand for acute care beds prompted Summa Health System to improve its process for transfers between long-term and acute care. Summa Health System partnered with long-term care professionals in its service area to establish the Care Coordination Network (CCN). Agencies included 28 skilled nursing facilities, local EMS/ambulance providers, and the local Area Agency on Aging. The CCN began by establishing a Memorandum of Understanding in acceptance of the goals to improve patient outcomes. Specific goals included the following:

- Improve access to skilled nursing beds for Summa Health System patients

- Improve the transition process between acute and long-term care, including communication and coordination

- Take advantage of the combined resources to effectively manage healthcare resources and improve clinical care, including optimizing the expertise present at all levels of care

Because communication issues led the list of concerns for all participants, the CCN first adopted a consistent nursing facility referral process, which included guidelines for determining postacute care needs and procedures for discussing them with patients. To standardize communication, the CCN also adopted a single, postacute transfer form. An electronic referral process was implemented, which allowed CCN members to query each other regarding bed availability, patient needs, and other transition issues. In addition, outcomes measures were developed to track the success of the processes and their impact on patient care.

Program outcomes for the 3,000 patients discharged to postacute care have been positive for Summa Health System. Over the initial three-year period, 31-day readmission rates decreased from 26% to 24%, and average length of stay decreased from 7.4 to 7.1 days. These improvements allowed Summa Health System to increase its volume by 130 patients without adding resources, and decrease its hours on emergency department diversion. Appointments for one-day surgery and follow-up testing also were kept more frequently because instructions were more consistently communicated.

The process for collaboration is described online, and access to the group's transfer form is provided. The process for collaboration among more than 30 organizations is instructive for anyone attempting to bring together diverse interests to tackle a complex issue. The transfer form is worth evaluating for adoption or modification to an organization's specifications.[12]

INTERACT II (Working Together to Improve Care and Reduce Acute Care Transfers)

INTERACT II (Working Together to Improve Care and Reduce Acute Care Transfers) is a toolkit designed for nursing homes to reduce hospital transfers. The toolkit includes materials designed to help you do the following:

- Identify early changes in clinical status

- Comprehensively assess the resident once a clinical change has been noted

- Document clinical status changes

- Communicate more effectively with the clinical team regarding status changes

Background

The Georgia Medical Care Foundation, the Medicare Quality Improvement Organization (QIO) for the state of Georgia, designed the first iteration of the INTERACT program with three participating nursing homes that had high rates of hospitalizations. The program was developed through a prospective quality improvement process that included providing participating nursing homes with communication and clinical practice tools, as well as telephonic support from a nurse practitioner.

INTERACT prevented avoidable hospital admissions in the three nursing homes participating in the pilot study, but, given the small convenience sample, Ouslander and colleagues concluded further study was needed. A study funded with a grant from the Commonwealth Fund is in process and is expected to end in July 2010; however, the toolkit has been refined and is available online. Many nursing homes are using the refined version, INTERACT II. We will follow a nursing home patient through the INTERACT II process to take a closer look at the toolkit.

The INTERACT II toolkit
The Early Warning Tool

Use of the INTERACT II tools begins when the nursing home staff notices a change in the resident's status. The Early Warning Tool is to be completed by anyone having direct care responsibility for the resident during or at the end of a shift. This is generally the certified nursing assistant (CNA), and the report is made to the nurse. The purpose of the Early Warning Tool is to:

- Identify and document changes in resident status

- Communicate changes to other members of the clinical team

Its regular use should improve resident care and proactively treat issues that could result in an acute care transfer if left unattended.

The elements of the Early Warning Tool follow the acronym "Stop and Watch":

- **S**eems different than usual

- **T**alks or communicates less than usual

- **O**verall, needs more help than usual

- **P**articipates in activities less than usual

- **A**te less than usual (not because of dislike of food)

- N

- Drank less than usual

- Weight change

- Agitated or nervous more than usual

- Tired, weak, confused, or drowsy

- Change in skin color or condition

- Help with walking, transferring, toileting more than usual

Let's follow Mrs. J, her CNA, Margaret, and her nurse, Mike.

Mrs. J has been a resident in Shadyside Nursing Home for two years. She has a history of congestive heart failure, atrial fibrillation, and total joint disease. A social person, Mrs. J has many friends at Shadyside and can often be found in any of the community-gathering spaces playing cards, working at crafts, or simply visiting with the other residents. Mrs. J has a son and daughter who live in the area and visit often.

Upon arriving for her afternoon shift, Margaret discovers that Mrs. J has not been out of her room all day. Because this is not typical, Margaret makes it a priority to check with her. Margaret's visit with Mrs. J yields information that is concerning. Mrs. J is not as talkative or as active as usual and she seems a little confused. Mrs. J tells Margaret that she has lower abdominal tenderness and often feels like she has to use the bathroom. Margaret records this information in the Early Warning Form and reports these changes to the nurse, Mike, who decides to follow the care path: Symptoms for Urinary Tract Infection (UTI).

Care paths and change in condition cards

The INTERACT II toolkit includes care paths and change in condition reference cards for some common conditions experienced by frail older adults that often result in acute care transfers. They are designed to be used primarily by licensed care staff but can also be used by physicians, NPs, and physician assistants (PA). The care paths are set up like flow charts that guide the assessment process. The flow chart begins with the assessment and takes the nurse through assessment of vital signs, notification of the physician (or NP/PA), request and evaluation of laboratory testing, and, finally, transfer to the hospital or continuing management at the skilled nursing facility. Care paths are included for mental status change, fever, lower respiratory infection, congestive heart failure, UTI, and dehydration. The goals of the care paths and condition reference cards are to:

+ Provide evidence-based guidance on the management of common conditions in the skilled nursing facility

+ Facilitate timely, effective communication with members of the treatment team

Let's check in with Mrs. J to see how these tools are used.

Mike takes Mrs. J's vital signs; she has a temperature of 102.5°F, and her heartbeat and respirations are 110 and 40, respectively. In addition, Mrs. J hasn't eaten much all day. Mike documents his findings using the SBAR (Situation, Background, Assessment/Appearance, and Recommendation) communication tool and contacts the nurse practitioner, Denise.

SBAR

The SBAR tool helps to improve communication between the treatment team by providing guidelines that ensure all members are using consistent language. This tool is used any time the resident experiences a change in condition and it is necessary to call the physician, NP, or PA. In addition, it is used for shift-to-shift communication among nursing staff.

The SBAR framework includes Situation, Background, Assessment (for RNs) or Appearance (for LPNs), and Recommendation. When providing information about the situation, the nurse should concisely describe the problem, when it started, and any interventions that make the problem better or worse. Background should include the resident's primary diagnosis (or reason for being in the nursing home), pertinent medical history, mental status or neurological changes, vital signs, pain level, changes in function and nutritional status, changes in skin color and wound status, laboratory values, medication changes or medical orders in the last two weeks, advance directives, and allergies. Assessment information includes a brief description of what the nurse thinks is going on with the resident. This can be the identification of the care plan being followed. Finally, the nurse makes a specific request for a provider visit, additional testing, a change in medication or other orders, IV or SC fluids, or continued monitoring of vital signs. Let's see what Denise decides to do with Mrs. J.

Denise orders a urinalysis, a culture and sensitivity, a complete blood count, and a basic metabolic panel. She then assesses Mrs. J and finds she meets the criteria for beginning antibiotics immediately. Denise orders the antibiotics and asks Mike to monitor Mrs. J's vital signs every four hours and report any changes. When the laboratory values return, Denise finds Mrs. J did have a UTI, so the antibiotics are continued.

Mrs. J met the criteria and was treated successfully in the nursing home. If the resident met the criteria for an acute care transfer, the process would have continued with completion of additional forms, transfer of important documentation, and a quality review.

Mrs. J—INTERACT Strategies

- Investigate any atypical behaviors and symptoms. Document and report them.

- Follow the appropriate care path

- Communicate interventions using SBAR

Resident Transfer Form

Once the decision has been made to transfer the patient to the hospital, the nurse at the long-term care facility completes the Resident Transfer Form and puts it in a specially marked envelope with all pertinent documentation. The Resident Transfer Form is to be completed for each acute care transfer and includes the following information:

- The name of the nursing home and hospital

- The name, date of birth, and primary language of the resident

- The status of the resident, either short-term or long-term rehabilitation

- The resident's primary contact person, their healthcare proxy status, and whether they are aware of the diagnosis and acute care transfer

- The resident's code status

- Contact information for the referring provider and other nursing home contact

- The reason for the transfer

- Baseline mental and functional status

- Identification of devices or special treatments

- Risk alerts, such as pressure ulcers, aspiration or wandering, and isolation precautions

- Capability of the nursing home to care for conditions such as IV therapy

- Conditions under which the nursing home would accept this patient back

- Skin care needed

- Immunizations

- Diet

+ Physical therapy and capability related to ADL

+ Continence, disabilities, or impairments

+ Behavioral or social issues

+ Pain assessment

+ The reason for the original long-term care admission and whether there is a bed hold in place

The purpose of the Resident Transfer Form is to ensure a safe handoff to the emergency department by providing essential information that will lead to an appropriate evaluation of the resident.

The Resident Transfer Form is not meant to repeat information documented elsewhere. Additional documentation is included in a specially marked envelope. The envelope contains a listing of the documentation included. Documentation that must always accompany the patient include the following:

+ Resident Transfer Form and face sheet

+ Current medication list or medication administration record

+ Advance directives, DNR status, and care-limiting orders

+ The bed-hold policy

+ Optional documentation includes:

+ The SBAR form or nurse's progress note

+ Most recent history and physical and any recent discharge summary

+ Recent providers' orders related to the acute condition

+ Relevant lab results and x-rays

+ A listing of personal belongings being sent with the patient

The listing printed on the envelope is intended to ensure a systematic gathering of all pertinent information and ensure that essential information is located in one easily recognizable place.

Continuous learning and quality improvement

Within 24 to 48 hours of the acute care transfer, the long-term care facility can conduct an assessment to review the acute care transfer and facilitate continuous learning and quality improvement. The quality review includes identification of the reason for the acute care transfer and any other hospitalizations the resident has experienced in the past year; the clinical scenario using the SBAR form and progress notes; and prompts for assessing whether the acute care transfer could have been avoided. A quality improvement review should be conducted on two to three acute care transfers per week so that patterns can be identified and analyzed.

Advance care planning tools

The INTERACT II toolkit also includes a framework for advance care planning. The Communication Guide covers suggestions for starting and conducting the conversation about advance care planning. It includes techniques for establishing trust and communicating with compassion, and offers scripted language for discussing end-of-life care. Finally, this part of the toolkit includes characteristics of residents likely to be entering the active dying process and a listing of comfort care interventions.

The purpose of the advance care tools is to provide guidance for what is often a difficult conversation with residents and their families. The overarching goal is to provide residents with comfort and dignity when they are in the active dying process.

The Champion

Implementation of the INTERACT II toolkit is facilitated by a Champion. The Champion is charged with educating all staff about the tools and coaching staff in their use. As the name implies, Champions drive the implementation of this program by planning the implementation and constantly solving issues that arise so that the process isn't sidetracked. Communication about the use of the INTERACT II toolkit with residents is encouraged.[13]

Expected outcomes and further study

Ouslander and colleagues compiled outcomes of the original 18-month pilot. They included staff satisfaction with the toolkit and an analysis of preventable hospitalizations. A major finding was related to potentially preventable acute care transfers.

Although rates of hospitalization varied widely among the participating nursing homes, 40% were considered preventable. During the six-month study period, readmissions declined by 50%, and those admissions rated as potentially avoidable decreased from 77% to 49%.

Staff satisfaction with the toolkit was high, although none of the nursing homes implemented all of the tools. Ouslander concluded that, in order to implement the toolkit, an infrastructure must be built so that the tools become part of everyday practice. Further, he believes the intervention developed shows promise but must be subjected to further testing before results can be generalized, given the small convenience sample in the pilot study.[14]

The toolkit is in the process of being refined, and the program (INTERACT II) is being studied with a larger and more diverse sample of nursing homes. This follow-up study is being funded with a grant from the Commonwealth Fund and will conclude in July 2010. Study outcomes include use of the toolkit, hospitalization rates, and the cost of the intervention.[15] The toolkit and detailed instructions for use are available online for leaders interested in adoption.

Additional Factors Affecting Acute Care Transfers

It should be noted that other system factors affecting acute care transfers have been identified and are generally system issues. These include bed-hold policies and per diem rates. Intrator and colleagues found the presence of a bed-hold policy increased the likelihood of acute care transfers, whereas per diem rates tended to discourage this practice.[16]

Grabowsi and colleagues studied predictors of acute care transfers and found them related to resident's welfare and preferences, provider attitudes, and financial considerations. Factors related to the resident's welfare included sociodemographics, health characteristics, nurse staffing, the presence of ancillary services, and the use of hospice services. Factors associated with increased rates of hospitalization included resident preferences and provider concerns about issues like overburdened staff at the nursing home.[17]

Final Thoughts

Anyone who has worked to improve transitions between nursing homes and hospitals would be impressed by the programs emerging to address these issues. Underlying all of these programs is the relationship among the professional care staff on behalf of patients. The term "healthcare system" implies a coordinated framework driven by a common goal; however, silos exist perpetuated by payment structures. The recent changes related to bundling will have a profound effect on all of that, and those of us in the trenches will be scrambling to respond. If prospective payment taught us anything, it is that the great minds in healthcare will figure out how to improve on behalf of the patients we serve. If we are to do it right, we will have to build mutual trust and respect. As Kyle Allen, DO, told the CCN, "Leave your competition at the door; this is about improving quality."[18]

References

1. O. Intrator, D.C. Grabowski, J. Zinn, M. Schleinitz, Z. Feng, S. Miller, V. Mor, "Hospitalization of Nursing Home Residents: The Effects of States' Medicaid Payment and Bed-Hold Policies," *Health Services Research*. 42 (2007): 1651–71.

2. K.M. Terrell, D.K. Miller, "Critical Review of Transitional Care Between Nursing Homes and Emergency Departments," *Annals of Long Term Care* Vol 15: 2 Feb 01, 2007.

3. M.N. Davis, S.T. Smith, S. Tyler, "Improving Transition and Communication Between Acute Care and Long-Term Care: A System for Better Continuity of Care," *Annals of Long Term Care*, Vol 13: 5 May 01, 2005.

4. E.A. Coleman, P.D. Fox, "One Patient, Many Places: Managing Health Care Transitions, Part I: Introduction, Accountability, Information for Patients in Transition," Vol 12: 9 Sept 1, 2004

5. R.L. Kane, G. Keckhafer, S. Flood, B. Bershadsky, M.S. Siadaty, "The Effect of Evercare on Hospital Use," *Journal of American Geriatrics Society*, 51 (2003): 1427–34.

6. E. Hutt, M. Ecord, T.B. Eilertsen, E. Frederickson, A.M. Kramer, "Precipitants of Emergency Room Visits and Acute Hospitalization in Short-Stay Medicare Nursing Home Residents," *Journal of American Geriatrics Society*, 50 (2002): 223–9.

7. M.D. Naylor, E.T. Kurtzman, M.V. Pauly. "Transitions of Elders between Long-Term Care and Hospitals," *Policy, Politics, & Nursing Practice* 10 (2009): 187–94. Epub 2009 Dec 20.

8. See note 5 above.

9. H. Gravelle, M. Dusheiko, R. Sheaff, P. Sargent, R. Boaden, S. Pickard, et al., "Impact of Case Management (Evercare) on Frail Elderly Patients: Controlled before and after Analysis of Quantitative Outcome Data," *BMJ* 2007 January 6; 334(7583): 31. Published online 2006 November 15. DOI: 10.1136/bmj.39020.413310.55.

10. R. Sheaff, R. Boaden, P. Sargent, S. Pickard, H. Gravelle, S. Parker S, et al., "Impacts of Case Management for Frail Elderly People: A Qualitative Study," *Journal of Health Services Research & Policy*, 14 (2009): 88–95.

11. See note 9 above.

12. D. McCarthy, C. Beck, "Summa Health System's Care Coordination Network," The Commonwealth Fund. August 2007.

13. INTERACT II Resource Binder: Working Together to Improve Care, Communication, and Continuity for our Residents. May 2009

14. J.G. Ouslander, M. Perloe, J.H. Givens, L. Kluge, T. Rutland, G. Lamb. Reducing potentially avoidable hospitalizations of nursing home residents: results of a pilot quality improvement project. *J Am Med Dir Assoc*. 2009 Nov;10(9): 644-52. Epub 2009 Oct 12.

15. J. Ouslander, *Reducing Avoidable Hospitalizations of Nursing Home Residents: Refinement and Evaluation of a Toolkit for Nursing Home Health Professionals*, accessed April 17, 2010 *www.commonwealthfund.org/Content/Grants/2008/Aug/Reducing-Avoidable-Hospitalizations-of-Nursing-Home-Residents--Refinement-and-Evaluation-of-a-Toolki.aspx*.

16. See note 1 above.

17. D.C. Grabowski, K.A. Stewart, S.M. Broderick, L.A. Coots, "Predictors of Nursing Home Hospitalization: A Review of the Literature," *Medical Care Research and Review*, 65 (2008): 3–39.

18. See note 12 above.

Culturally Competent Transitions

LEARNING OBJECTIVES

After reading this chapter, you should be able to:

- Define cultural and linguistic competence and outline its impact on healthcare organizations

- Identify mandated and suggested standards for providing culturally competent care

Thus far, we have treated all patients as though they have the same basic cultural underpinnings and will respond to our efforts in a homogenous fashion. Although this was appropriate for our early discussions on transitions programming, an exploration of the impact of culture is necessary given our increasingly diverse patient population.

Chronic Disease: A Cultural Issue?

It is estimated that by 2050, almost half of the U.S. population will be made up of ethnic and racial minorities.[1]

It is imperative to ensure culture is addressed in transitions programming. The incidence of morbidity from chronic illness is higher in racial and ethnic minorities.[2] Among adults age 50 and older, African Americans and Latinos are more likely than whites to have at least one of the most common chronic conditions: asthma, cancer, heart disease, diabetes, high blood pressure, obesity, or anxiety/depression.[3] African Americans and American Indians/Alaska Natives are more likely to be limited in activities of daily living because of a chronic condition.[4]

As we have discussed, one of the most frequent causes of hospital readmission is lack of timely follow-up with an appropriate physician. Racial and ethnic minorities are less likely to have a physician who is providing regular care. Further, language barriers are problematic, since most of the patient education and coaching provided is language-based and in English. Perhaps that is one reason that racial and ethnic minorities do not feel like a partner with healthcare providers and report less participation in medical decisions.[5] Not surprisingly, racial and ethnic minorities are much more likely to be dissatisfied with healthcare.[6]

Organizational Commitment to Cultural Competence

Fortunately, the commitment to providing culturally competent care seems to be growing among healthcare organizations. The impetus could be to address the mandate of Healthy People 2010 to eliminate racial and ethnic disparities, or perhaps it is other state or federal guidelines. Or, it could be that it is simply good business practice to address the needs of the local community.[7] Whatever the reason, there seems to be a growing interest in providing culturally competent healthcare.

Cultural and linguistic competence has been defined by the U.S. Department of Health and Human Services (HHS) as

> *A set of congruent behaviors, attitudes, and policies that come together in a system, agency, or among professionals that enables effective work in cross-cultural situations. 'Culture' refers to integrated patterns of human behavior that include the language, thoughts, communications, actions, customs, beliefs, values, and institutions of racial, ethnic, religious, or social groups. 'Competence' implies having the capacity to function effectively as an individual and an organization within the context of the cultural beliefs, behaviors, and needs presented by consumers and their communities.*[8]

Further, HHS has set forth 14 standards for Culturally and Linguistically Appropriate Services (CLAS). Four of these standards (standards 4–7) are mandates for all recipients of federal funds (**Figure 8.1** lists the non-mandatory standards).

Standard 4: Healthcare organizations must offer and provide language assistance services, including bilingual staff and interpreter services, at no cost to each patient/consumer with limited English proficiency at all points of contact, in a timely manner during all hours of operation.

Standard 5: Healthcare organizations must provide to patients/consumers in their preferred language both verbal offers and written notices informing them of their right to receive language assistance services.

Standard 6: Healthcare organizations must ensure the competence of language assistance provided to limited English proficient patients/consumers by interpreters and bilingual staff. Family and friends should not be relied on to provide interpretation services (except on request by the patient/consumer).

Standard 7: Healthcare organizations must make available easily understood patient-related materials and post signage in the languages of the commonly encountered groups and/or groups represented in the service area.[9]

These are minimum standards, and most healthcare organizations have been doing these things for years. The CLAS Standards National Project Advisory Committee also makes more challenging, and one might argue, meaningful recommendations.

First, the standards seem to set forth a guiding principle that all patients receive effective, understandable, and respectful care that is provided in a manner congruent with their cultural beliefs and primary language. Related to this, CLAS also directs that all healthcare staff should be trained in culturally appropriate skills. The Committee recommends that organizations hire, retain, and promote a diverse workforce in order to have a healthcare workforce representing the communities they serve.

CLAS makes recommendations regarding how organizations approach this issue strategically, and suggests a baseline assessment of cultural and linguistic competence. This assessment should include a cultural profile of the community. This can form the basis for a strategic plan, which the Committee recommends to set forth clear goals, policies, operational plans, and accountability. Performance measures for the organization and for individual staff should be included.

Once the planning of improvement activities begins, CLAS recommends involving a culturally diverse group of patients in planning and designing services. Specific activities could include documenting cultural and linguistic preferences in patients' medical records and implementing grievance procedures. Finally, healthcare organizations should make their commitment to cultural and linguistic competence public.[10]

Figure 8.1

Culturally and Linguistically Appropriate Services (CLAS)— Nonmandatory Standards

1	Culturally competent care should be provided.
2	Healthcare organizations should implement practices that recruit, retain and promote a workforce reflective of its geographic area.
3	All staff should receive training to promote cultural competence.
8	Healthcare organizations should have a strategic plan for ensuring cultural competence.
9	Healthcare organizations should continually assess their cultural competence.
10	Cultural, ethnic and linguistic preferences of patients should be collected and recorded.
11	A profile of the community should be maintained.
12	The community should be involved in designing and implementing CLAS activities.
13	Conflict and grievance processes should be culturally and linguistically sensitive.
14	Healthcare organizations should make their CLAS activities public.

Healthcare organizations can evaluate their cultural competence with the Organizational Cultural Competence Assessment Profile, developed by The Lewin Group, Inc. for the Health Resources and Services Administration. This assessment helps organizations identify and evaluate their approach to the critical elements for measuring cultural competence.[11]

Cultural Competence and Transitions

The National Transitions of Care Coalition used the Cultural Competence standards set forth by the National Association of Social Work to develop strategies for ensuring culturally competent transitions.

Standard 1: Ethics and Values

Cultural and linguistic competence is compatible with self-management and patient empowerment, the cornerstones of transitional care. To participate fully on the healthcare team, patients must be understood, culturally and linguistically.

Strategies related to this standard include adhering to professional ethics and values, while recognizing when these professional codes conflict with cultural competence. The National Transitions of Care Coalition also recommends referring to United Nations conventions and declarations to receive a global context.

Standard 2: Self-Awareness

One of the best ways to increase your appreciation of others' cultural identities is to develop an awareness of your own values, beliefs, and biases. Do some soul-searching. Think about your culture and assess how it may influence your views about people with different cultural backgrounds. Educate yourself about how fear, ignorance, and systematic oppression can influence the way people behave toward one another in a healthcare setting. Make an honest evaluation about whether your beliefs have influenced your professional practice.

Standard 3: Cross-Cultural Knowledge

Developing cultural competency is truly a continuing education process. It may require frequent relearning and unlearning about diversity. Healthcare professionals should continuously expand their knowledge related to the various cultural groups they serve. Although it is important to acknowledge differences among groups, you should also recognize individual differences within those groups to avoid stereotyping. Continuously develop your knowledge base of cultural characteristics and how they affect behaviors and perceptions related to health, illness, healthcare services, disability, caregiving, death, and dying.

Standard 4: Cross-Cultural Skills

Cross-cultural knowledge is exhibited when cross-cultural skills are employed. These skills include the following:

- Techniques used by healthcare professionals should reflect knowledge related to the impact of culture on helping processes.

- Healthcare professionals should engage patients by exhibiting warmth, genuineness, empathy, openness, and flexibility.

- Healthcare professionals must identify culturally normative and symptomatic behaviors and recognize both strengths and potential weaknesses when assessing the cultural impact on health and function.

- Communication regarding cultural groups should emphasize strengths rather than limitations.

Standard 5: Culturally and Linguistically Appropriate Service Delivery

This standard speaks to the healthcare delivery system and the need to put in place organizational structures for cultural competence. In addition to making sure all staff is educated, organizations should engage patients from culturally diverse backgrounds in developing and evaluating the organization's programming. To ensure organizational support at all levels, cultural competence should be included in the mission, vision, and goals. And community resources that support the cultural needs of the population should be utilized effectively on behalf of patients.

Standard 6: Workforce

One of the best ways to ensure cultural and linguistic competence is to ensure the organization reflects its community. Strategies include those targeted at hiring, promotion, and retention practices that encourage diversity. Further, all staff should be encouraged to develop expertise in cultural and linguistic skills.

Standard 7: Advocacy

Beyond adopting practices as individuals, healthcare professionals and their organizations can advocate for improvements to the healthcare system overall. Healthcare organizations can partner with other advocacy groups to cause change in public policy to promote cultural and linguistic competence.[12]

A Broad View

As we close this discussion on cultural and linguistic competence, I would like to encourage you to view culture broadly. It is more than ethnic diversity. For example, the deaf community can be culturally defined and served, and deaf patients who sign are very similar to those who speak foreign languages, in terms of syntax and grammar. Also, the LGBT (Lesbian, Gay, Bisexual, and Transgender) community has characteristics and preferences related to healthcare with which it would behoove us to familiarize ourselves. Recognizing cultural backgrounds while being mindful of the individualism within groupings will help us to provide respectful care to all of our patients.

References

1. J.C. Day, *Population Projections of the United States by Age, Sex, Race, and Hispanic Origin: 1995 to 2050* (U.S. Bureau of the Census, Current Population Reports, Washington DC: U.S. Government Printing Office, 1996).

2. E. Ihara, *Cultural Competence in Health Care: Is it Important for People with Chronic Conditions?* (Washington DC: Center on an Aging Society: Georgetown University, 2004).

3. K.H. Collins, *Diverse Communities, Common Concerns: Assessing Health Care Quality for Minority Americans*, (New York: The Commonwealth Fund, 2002).

4. V.M. Fried, *Health, United States, 2003: Chartbook on Trends in the Health of Americans*, (Hyattsville, MD: National Center for Health Statistics, 2003).

5. L.A. Cooper, "Patient-Provider Communication: The Effect of Race and Ethnicity on Process and Outcomes of Healthcare," In S. A. Smedley BD, *Unequal Treatment: Confronting Racial and Ethnic Disparities in Health Care*, (Washington, DC: The National Academies Press, 2003), 552–593.

6. See note 2 above.

7. See note 2 above.

8. CLAS Standards National Project Advisory Committee. (2001). *National Standards for Culturally and Linguistically Appropriate Services in Health Care: Final Report*, (Washington DC: U.S. Department of Health and Human Services, OPHS; Office of Minority Health).

9. See note 8 above.

10. See note 8 above.

11. K.W. Linkins, (2002). *Indicators of Cultural Competence in Health Care Delivery Organizations: An Organizational Cultural Competence Assessment Profile*, (Washington DC: The Health Resources and Services Administration; U.S. Department of Health and Human Services).

12. National Transitions of Care Coalition, *Cultural Competence: Essential Ingredient for Successful Transitions of Care.* Retrieved May 13, 2010, from National Transitions of Care Coalition: (2008–2010), *www.ntocc.org/Portals/0/ CulturalCompetence.pdf.*

Pulling It All Together

At this point, if I have done my job, many of these programs sound like they would be perfect for adoption at your hospital. So, is it possible to implement all of them and create some synergistic benefit? If you are interested in tackling your inpatient discharge process, as well as transitional care for both community dwellers and nursing home patients, it seems like these programs could complement one another. A word of caution, however: Each of these programs represents such a different paradigm for most healthcare providers, that easing into the change by implementing one program at a time seems like the wisest approach. Healthcare leaders will need to evaluate their own situation and decide on the best course. The following discussion on a total approach should be helpful in stimulating your thought process.

A Total Approach

The Commonwealth Fund recently released a report that provides a brief overview of many programs designed to reduce readmissions and which part of the continuum the programs would address—during the hospitalization, at the time of discharge, or after discharge. The Fund also includes its assessment of the implementation complexity associated with each program.

Many of the recommendations related to inpatient hospitalization focus on improving communication and collaboration between the treatment team in the hospital and the clinical professionals who will pick up care after the hospitalization. Also included is a recommendation to assess risk at the time of hospitalization. This identifies specific issues so intervention can be tailored to the individual needs of the highest-risk patients. There seems to be recognition that improvement is needed in the one-size-fits-all approach long used in hospital discharge planning.

The report's recommendation regarding teaching method is the teach back approach. This method is a good, basic start that is easy to implement. It recognizes that the patient nodding his head yes may not necessarily understand what he is hearing. The teach back approach involves asking the patient to repeat the information he just received. Including the adult learning principles and checking for understanding, and not only imitation, would enhance this recommendation.

The last recommendation related to the hospitalization includes attempting to learn about the patient's wishes regarding end-of-life planning so that advance care planning is discussed across the continuum.

The recommendations at discharge relate to those elements identified as a frequent cause of readmissions. The report emphasizes medication reconciliation and education and a follow-up physician appointment. Also recommended is a mechanism to ensure patient understanding of the discharge instructions, including what to do if there is a problem, and identification of pending test results. Following national guidelines and clinical pathways for discharge plans, as well as ensuring timely communication with the next provider, are recommendations directed toward physicians, specifically. The recommendations for nursing home transfers are to use a standard form to enhance communication and a nurse practitioner to provide treatment in the nursing home.

Probably the most transformational recommendations are related to the post-discharge phase. The over-arching recommendation seems to be for the hospital to continue to take responsibility for patient self-management after he leaves the hospital proper. The personal health record (PHR) is the tool suggested for recordkeeping. Home visits, follow-up phone calls, and the use of Telehealth in homecare are specific recommended interventions. Accomplishing this through community partnerships is emphasized.[1]

Components of a Total Approach

A complete approach to managing hospital readmissions that would address the recommendations made by the Commonwealth Fund could include all of the programs discussed, implemented as an integrated process (**see Figure 9.1**). The resultant process would maximize patient self-management and smooth transitions, ultimately minimizing the potential for a readmission. Whether the clinician facilitating the process and providing support was a transitional care nurse, discharge advocate, or transition coach would be a strategic decision based on a hospital's needs, goals, and resource limitations.

Figure 9.1

The Total Approach for Hospitals

Assess Risk	Transitional Care Model – rehospitalization risk factors
	Patient Activation Measure – knowledge, skill and confidence
	Newest Vital Sign – health literacy
Prepare Patient for Discharge	RED – organize the discharge elements following national guidelines
	Care Transitions Intervention[SM] Pillars—begin using PHR, Medications, Red Flags
Transition Patient Home	Care Transitions Intervention[SM]—home and phone visits to continue work on the pillars and enable self management
	Transitional Care – physician, home and phone visits to enable patient self management
Transition Patient to the Nursing Home	SUMMA's Care Coordination Network – collaborate with nursing home clinicians to develop effective communication methods
	INTERACT – collaborate with nursing home clinicians to develop care pathways that provide seamless transfers

Assessing risk

The first stage of the process could be to assess patient risk using criteria developed by Mary Naylor, PhD, RN. According to Naylor, a patient is at risk of readmission if he meets two or more of the following criteria:

- Is age 80 or older

- Has moderate to severe functional deficits

- Has an active behavioral and/or psychiatric health issue

- Has four or more active co-existing health conditions

- Has six or more prescribed medications

- Has had two or more hospitalizations within the past six months

- Was hospitalized within the past 30 days

- Has inadequate support systems

- Has low health literacy

- Has a documented history of nonadherence to the therapeutic regimen

In addition to this assessment, the patient's health literacy level is evaluated using the Newest Vital Sign™, and the patient's readiness for self-management is assessed using the Patient Activation Measure (PAM).

The assessment conducted could affect decisions related to after-hospital care and support services. It would also help the treatment team target the patient education provided related to literacy level and readiness for self-management. Adult education principles should form the foundation for education content development and delivery.

The inpatient interdisciplinary team

RED is the discharge process hospitalized patients would experience in this total approach. The team implements a systematic process for ensuring the discharge plan based on national guidelines and care plans. They verify and reconcile medications. In addition, the interdisciplinary team has a formal process for keeping each other informed about plans and further information relating to discharge.

Following this process, the patient is educated about his or her discharge plan, test results available after discharge, and medications. Patient education materials containing consistent information, meaningful for patients with low health literacy, are used. Appointments for physician follow-up and outpatient tests or treatments are coordinated with the patient and scheduled, and there is a discussion about procedures for handing unanticipated issues. A hospital employee functioning in a discharge advocate (DA) role coordinates the discharge on behalf of the interdisciplinary treatment team and functions as a contact support person for the patient so questions and difficulties related to discharge are addressed.

Then, a follow-up appointment is scheduled for the patient, and a comprehensive discharge summary and medication list is expedited to the physician.

Incorporate self-management and transitional care into the hospital stay

The Care Transitions Intervention^{SM} pillars are fundamental to any program intended to manage transitions and encourage patient self-management. The pillars begin during the hospitalization and continue throughout the transition. The RED patient education materials include content similar to that covered in the Care Transitions Intervention, so unifying the two should not be difficult.

Patients begin by establishing a personal goal while in the hospital. They also begin to complete a PHR and a personal medication record. The hospital staff person functioning in the transition coach role would review the red flags. This would be similar to the discussion a discharge advocate would have with the patient regarding his primary diagnosis.

The DA and transition coach roles could be blended in the hospital because much of the same content is included in the RED and Care Transitions Intervention programs. A word of caution, however: The focus of the transition coach is to encourage the *patient* to solve problems, ask questions, and so on. While in the hospital, the DA solves discharge-related problems and coordinates care. It can be difficult for the same person to fluctuate between the doing role and the coaching role. The right person may be able to manage it by teaching the patient to take the opportunity, while in the hospital, to advocate, provide information, and ask questions.

Coordinating care and solving problems would happen behind the scenes while the patient is in the hospital. Once the patient is discharged, the DA or transition coach needs to stop doing things for the patient and adopt a purely coaching role.

After hospitalization

If you are following the Care Transitions Intervention, there is one visit at home. If you are following the Transitional Care Program, visits after the hospitalization include accompanying the patient to physician visits and visiting with the patient at home. The precise number of visits is determined by the advance practice nurse.

The home visit under the Care Transitions Intervention and the Transitional Care Program include a thorough review of medications. Medications prescribed upon discharge from the hospital are reviewed for accuracy and understanding. Often, patients leave the hospital with an adjusted dose for a medication they were already taking. This is frequently the cause of a medication discrepancy because patients revert to the old dose and never notice that it had been changed in the hospital.

During the home visit, patients are asked to collect all of the medications they take; this frequently includes medications that were never disclosed during the hospitalization. Patients do not always realize they are supposed to tell the nurse at the hospital about all of the over-the-counter and herbal medicines they were taking. Moreover, sometimes patients simply forget, especially if their medication regime is complex. Patients will complete the personal medication record once all of the medications have been collected.

The personal medication record is also updated, and patients are encouraged to bring this record to every medical visit. The red flags for their chronic conditions are reviewed. Special emphasis is placed on how to stay healthy and what to do if their condition deteriorates. The transition coach ensures the patient understands how to access care. This could include role-playing or having the patient make a phone call under the watchful eye of the coach.

Finally, the transition coach or transitional care nurse makes sure the patient has follow-up appointments scheduled. If the appointments were not scheduled within an acceptable time frame, the coach may have the patient call to reschedule while the coach listens in and provides any necessary advice on how to handle scheduling difficulties.

Both the Care Transitions Intervention and the Transitional Care Program prepare patients for physician visits. The transition coach or transitional care nurse works with the patient to review expectations for the visit, coaches on how to achieve his objectives and how to get his most important questions answered, and instructs him to bring all of his medications.

The transitional care nurse would accompany the patient to the first physician appointment after discharge to facilitate understanding of the hospital discharge plan. The transitional care nurse may also advocate and facilitate on behalf of the patient in order to get all of his concerns addressed. If there is a need, the transitional care nurse may accompany the patient to more than one physician visit.

In the Transitional Care Program, the advance practice nurse continues to make home visits until they are no longer necessary. Both transition programs and the RED program include follow-up phone calls. The purpose of the phone calls in the RED program is to address issues related to medications and recent hospitalization. If transitional programming is implemented, a transition coach or transitional care nurse would do this during a home visit. The phone visits for transitions programming are for follow-up and reinforcement.

The process for nursing home patients

Nursing home patients or their caregivers receive education in the hospital related to chronic conditions, as well as medication indications and side effects. They may also benefit from coaching for self-advocacy. A great deal of attention should be placed on communication and collaboration between the treatment teams at the hospital and nursing home. The patient should feel the transition has been seamless and all clinical caregivers are on the same page. This seamlessness occurs with standardized information exchange, nurse-to-nurse reporting, and establishment of partnerships between hospital and nursing home providers.

The Process of Innovation

Implementing any of these innovative approaches to improving transitions and reducing readmissions will involve significant change for most organizations. According to Everett Rogers in his book, *Diffusion of Innovations*, innovation is "an idea, practice, or object that is perceived as new by an individual or other unit of adoption."[2] Many people resist innovation, even in healthcare, where change often seems to be the natural state. But, much has been written about processes for innovation that can inform the adoption of transition programming.

The environment for innovation

Most experts recommend beginning the process of implementing a new practice by analyzing the current environment in which the new process will function. Blanchard recommends both an assessment of the culture of an organization, overall, and an evaluation of the level of commitment by individuals.

Organizational culture is defined as the "predominant attitudes, beliefs, and behavior patterns that characterize an organization". If the hospital's culture is aligned with the goals and values of transitional programming, the existing culture can be leveraged to support the implementation. Historically, hospitals benefitted financially from readmissions. Therefore, there was no incentive to change and the culture may not have supported it. In addition, the culture at many healthcare organizations didn't support patient empowerment and self-management. A more paternalistic view reigned; we are here to take care of you, patient, and you just need to do what we tell you. If the culture and the change don't jibe, the foundational work of aligning them is necessary. Because of the revisions in the payment structure related to readmissions and bundling, hospitals should be motivated to align with these concepts.

On a more individual level, the commitment of the employees must be ascertained. New behaviors will most certainly be required based on the transitional programming. A great deal of work must be done to learn how committed the staff feel to the change.[3] Some staff members will embrace the new programming immediately, some will hold back until others get on board, some will resist until returning to the status quo is no longer an option, and some will never embrace the change. Rogers presents categories of adopters: innovators, early adopters, early majority, late majority, and laggards. These are ideal types, based on empirical evidence, which make comparison possible.

Innovators are characterized by an almost obsessively venturesome nature; they have a strong desire for the rash, the daring, and the risky. As such, they play a key role in the process of innovation by launching new ideas. Innovators have the ability to understand and apply complex knowledge. However, they must be able to cope with a high degree of uncertainty and the occasional setbacks that inevitably occur when introducing new ideas. It is helpful for the innovator to have control of resources to finance new ideas and absorb losses for those that aren't successful. The idea for transition programming would probably be brought to the institution by an innovator.

Early adopters are the group most respected by their peers. Because they are both willing to innovate and discrete about implementing new ideas, others look to early adopters for guidance during the diffusion of innovations. This group decreases uncertainty about new ideas by trying them and then sharing their subjective opinions with their interpersonal networks, who can then spread the findings. It may help to pilot transition programming on a unit led by an early adopter who can then provide his or her stamp of approval.

Representing approximately one third of the total group, the early majority adopts new ideas just ahead of the average. However, because they are between those who will adopt the idea early and those who will lag behind, the early majority provide an important link in the process. This group will deliberate for quite some time, but once they decide to support the new idea, they will do so purposefully. Although not generally thought of as opinion leaders, the early majority can help spread innovation by sheer numbers because they will interact often with their large peer group. It will be helpful to have a large percentage of the early majority on the unit piloting transition programming.

The late majority makes up another third of the total group and adopts innovation just after the average. This is a cautious group that will not adopt the innovation until most of the organization has already adopted the change and uncertainty about it has been eliminated. The late majority may be motivated to adopt the new transitions program by increasing economic or peer pressure.

Traditional in their views, laggards are the last to adopt innovation. This may be an entirely rational approach because the economic resources of laggards tend to be limited. As such, they must see that the innovation will not fail before they feel it is safe to adopt it. Existing staff members who are in this group may not apply for any of the positions in the transitions program until they are certain the program will succeed.[4]

Communication is necessary to bring people on board, but it can't be one-way communication. Leaders of the change must open themselves up to questions and concerns from staff. Staff members must feel free to express a dissenting view or question the change; it is the only way to rally people to the change. If staff is simply silenced into submission, they will never embrace the new program. Staff must be permitted to ask questions, mull over the idea, and express their concerns—and leaders should be prepared to address all of this. In working through this process with the staff, change leaders will bring people to a level of commitment that will enable the new process to become embedded into the culture of the organization.[5]

The future state

A clear and compelling picture of the future is an integral component of implementing innovation. The vision should describe a clear picture of the success created by implementing the change and allow individuals to see their success as a result of the change. It should also describe the urgency behind the change.[6]

Moreover, the vision should not be something that is developed and communicated with a top-down approach. In order for the change to be truly embedded in the organization, the vision must be shared among all stakeholders. Too often, a "vision statement" is either the result of the top leader's vision followed as long as the leader is in place, or it is the result of a crisis that binds everyone together for as long as the crisis lasts. In order to have vision that transcends any one person or situation, it must be shared throughout the organization. According to Senge:

> *A shared vision is not an idea. It is not even an important idea such as freedom. It is, rather, a force in people's hearts, a force of impressive power. It may be inspired by an idea, but once it goes further—if it is compelling enough to acquire the support of more than one person—then it is no longer an abstraction. It is palpable. People begin to see it as if it exists. Few, if any, forces in human affairs are as powerful as a shared vision. At its simplest level, a shared vision is the answer to the question, "What do we want to create?"*

There are techniques for creating a shared vision that can be studied and implemented. Basically, those desirous of implementing a change should enable each person to visualize their individual contribution to the change as a whole.[7]

Leading innovation

Any change initiative requires effective leadership. Particularly in these times of transformational change for healthcare, a new definition of leadership effectiveness is required. According to Senge, traditional leaders make key decisions and direct subordinates' participation. This type of leadership assumes the vision for the future, and talent to create it rests with the top of the organizational structure. This type of leadership can meet with short-term success as long as a charismatic leader is in place. Change that will outlast one leader must be embedded into the very fabric of the organization. Long-term, embedded change is accomplished through leadership characterized by supporting a vision shared by all staff. Leaders are stewards of a vision that represents a purpose they feel personally compelled to achieve. Leaders design systems that support the shared vision. And leaders teach, coach, and mentor staff rather than direct and coax.[8]

Leadership for implementing a change initiative should reside with a team made up of representatives who have a stake in the change. Members should represent each of the different viewpoints, including those who support, as well as those who question, the change. In order to be able to successfully implement the change process, leadership team members should be respected by their peers and have excellent communication and leadership skills.[9]

The change leadership team should have skills and knowledge that would contribute necessary expertise to planning for and implementing the change. A word of advice about who to invite: Although it doesn't make sense to pool ignorance, it is sometimes helpful to involve people who have the necessary talent and similar, but not exactly the same, experience. Sometimes, the best ideas for innovation come from people peripherally associated with the problem you are trying to solve. Being only indirectly involved, these individuals are able to see the problem with an open mind, unclouded by views taken for granted by people who have been enmeshed in the old way of doing things.

The team will facilitate, communicate, and design methods to set up the organization for success in implementing the change. A leadership team is responsible for the day-to-day roll out and should be able to communicate with one voice about the change.

The leadership team may consist of informal leaders, as well as those with formal leadership authority in the organization. If this is the case, the team facilitator must be skilled in leveling the playing field so that all team members feel valued and all input is given serious consideration by the group. Informal leaders can be important to the success of the change process because of their influence over stakeholder groups. In addition, they may have a point of view that the formal leaders in the organization do not realize; therefore, informal leaders can play a crucial part in the success or failure of the implementation of the transitions programming.

The innovation and leadership team must be supported by a sponsor. A sponsor is a senior leader who has the authority to remove organizational barriers and allocate necessary resources. The sponsor forms and formally charges the team, aligning it for success. Sponsors gain commitment to the change by encouraging concerns to surface and then addressing them, role-modeling behaviors expected of others, creating incentives for adopting the change, and fostering accountability to implement the change.[10]

The plan for innovation

Once the organization works through the process of developing a shared vision, led by the sponsor and change leadership team, all stakeholders should have a united view of what needs to be accomplished. The planning process can then take place. Again, it is useful to obtain information from as many stakeholders as possible in this process to ensure all contingencies have been taken into account. The planning process can begin by identifying a few key strategies and translating them into detailed implementation plans.[11]

Well-conceived implementation plans clarify priorities, provide enough information to get the implementation process started with the front line, and define desired outcomes. Part of the implementation plan can be to begin transition programming with a pilot to allow for experimentation on a small scale so rapid adjustments can be made, if necessary. This strategy can also enable the change team to have an early success to build upon.[12]

The roll out

Successful implementation of the transition program requires attention to budget, training, incentives, measuring results, and continual learning.

Budget

It is tempting for senior leaders to try to implement new initiatives with existing resources. In general, it is difficult to implement a major change initiative without investing in the infrastructure. Transitions programming is no exception. It is a setup for failure to ask staff to develop these innovations while continuing with their existing full-time responsibilities. Many of these programs can be implemented with a modest budget, but the change sponsor must approve some resources dedicated to the new transitions programming.[13]

Training

Most significant change initiatives require training to ensure the implementation staff have the necessary skill set for success.[14]

Transitions programming requires training in the roles of transition coach, transitional care nurse, DA, or Champion. The team working with this role will also need to be educated. Beyond that, organizations will benefit from training related to implementation of a major change initiative, including the topics addressed in this chapter. It is also helpful to have a mentor, someone who has implemented the transitions programming successfully. A mentor can provide advice regarding the inevitable unanticipated questions and issues that will arise during implementation.

Incentives

Incentives will help motivate the implementation staff, but this doesn't just refer to monetary incentives. Effective incentives can range from a simple "thank you" to a complex system based on goal achievement. Research shows that effective incentives are aligned with desired behaviors and the performance the innovation seeks to address. They must be made widely available to all involved with the change process, not just a select few. However, it is not necessary to over-incent this change process at the expense of other organizational goals.[15]

Performance measurement

Quality measures provide valuable information that will help all those involved track success, adjust when things aren't going as well as planned, identify areas of learning, and convince everyone involved to continue to support the change.

Donabedian defined a broadly supported approach to assessing quality measurement that includes the elements of structure, process, and outcome. Structure refers to the way a healthcare system is set up. Structure is important because it affects how people delivering care in the system behave. According to Donabedian, process measures can provide discriminating and valid judgments about care because those delivering care know processes contribute to their effectiveness. The advantages of process measures include the following:

- Ease of collection through relatively low-tech approaches, such as a check sheet or review of a medical record

- Immediate feedback related to whether the process is working

- The ability to discriminate small variations in quality

Outcomes are generally preferred as indicators of quality because the effect on the patient is what really matters. Although it is difficult to know that any one change process was independently the cause of an improvement in care, outcomes can reflect both what was done for a patient and the skill with which the care was delivered. In addition, patients can evaluate the effect of the outcome of care.[16]

Making it stick

This final element of implementation is often overlooked. It is important to the success of any change initiative to create accountability so that everyone involved in the change process, from the change leaders to implementation staff, knows his or her behavior is contributing to the success of the innovation. Characteristics of effective accountability include clearly defined and communicated indicators of success and regular checks on progress. It is important for everyone to be held accountable—leaders and frontline staff alike. In fact, leaders are probably the most closely watched of all. Everyone on the implementation team will take their cue from leadership. If the leaders' behaviors are in line with what they say is expected, frontline staff will take the change implementation more seriously.

Just keep swimming

In the animated movie, "Finding Nemo," Ellen DeGeneres' character, Dory, urges her partner on by singing, "Just keep swimming." This may be a good phrase to keep in mind as you move through the hurdles of establishing change. Implementing these innovations in healthcare will not proceed smoothly. There will be setbacks and frustrations, even in the most ideal environments. With a supportive change leadership team and staff who are willing to take a chance, you will succeed. The important thing is to track your progress, celebrate successes, and make any necessary adjustments. Try to plan for an early win; that should solidify everyone's support. And communicate far and wide about the important work you are doing.

References

1. The Commonwealth Fund, *Healthcare Leader Action Guide to Reduce Avoidable Readmissions* (Boston: The Commonwealth Fund, 2010).

2. E. Rogers, *Diffusion of Innovations*, Fifth Edition. (New York: Free Press, Simon & Schuster, 2003).

3. K. Blanchard, J. Britt, J. Hoekstra, P. Zigarmi, *Who Killed Change?* (New York: Harper Collins, 2009).

4. See note 2 above.

5. P. Senge, *The Fifth Discipline*, (New York: Doubleday, 1990).

6. See note 3 above.

7. See note 5 above.

8. See note 5 above.

9. See note 3 above.

10. See note 3 above.

11. C. Caldwell, D. Hutton, *Handbook for Managing Change in Healthcare*, (Milwaukee: Quality Press, 1998).

12. See note 3 above.

13. See note 3 above.

14. See note 11 above.

15. See note 3 above.

16. A. Donabedian, *The Definition of Quality and Approaches to its Assessment Vol 1. Explorations in Quality Assessment and Monitoring*, (Ann Arbor, Michigan: Health Administration Press, 1980).

APPENDIX

A Conversation With the Author

You have implemented transitional care programs following both the Coleman and Naylor Models and have led hospital departments responsible for discharge planning, so we'd like to talk about some of the lessons you learned along the way.

1. Why did you decide to implement transitions programs?

As the director of a geriatric service line, I noticed that we were expecting more and more from patients and their caregivers at home and the stress level was becoming intolerable for many of them. One of the volunteers at my hospital was a young 70-year-old retired teacher. She was a very bright, healthy, energetic woman. Her husband's health began to decline and he became very frail. He was often in and out of the hospital and she needed to stop volunteering. But I would see her often at the hospital and over time, she looked tired and more frail herself. I ran into her one day after she learned that she was going to be expected to take care of her husband's PICC line. She said, "I am so nervous. I'm not a nurse. How am I going to do this? I am so afraid I will hurt him." I will never forget those words or the emotion behind them. It was at that moment I knew we needed to do something different for patients and their families.

2. Were you concerned that you would just be adding another person to a team that was already providing discharge planning?

Our case managers were doing a heroic job of trying to make sure after-hospital care was arranged for each and every patient. And the bedside nurses were trying to make sure all of the discharge orders were written and review these orders with patients. But, in those processes, we weren't preparing patients and their families to self-manage. Patients were shaking their heads, saying, "Yes, I understand. I can do this." But, more and more of them were coming back with the same issues. Many were labeled "noncompliant." Preparing patients for self-management requires a different approach.

3. So, how is transitional care different from discharge planning?

Well, first of all the focus of transitional care is on self-management. The discharge arrangements are made and the discharge orders are established by the treatment team without necessarily knowing a great deal about what the patient and family can do. So, the focus of the transition coach or the transitional nurse is the patient and family and what they need to do after discharge. In getting to

A Conversation With the Author (cont.)

know what the family is currently doing at home, the transition coach (or transitional nurse) can provide valuable input into the discharge plan. But, she is not burdened by having to make all of those arrangements. In addition, the relationship with the patient and family continues into the home. I can't tell you how many things we learned about patients from spending some time in their homes. It is just not possible to learn about what is really happening related to self-care until you spend some time where it is happening.

Probably the most significant thing we learned about was the issue of health literacy. We had patients who were labeled "noncompliant" by their physicians and the physicians thought they were simply dealing with a patient who was recalcitrant. Once we saw what they were doing at home, it was obvious the issue was more one of health literacy. Once we provided the patient with education and tools, these patients miraculously became "compliant." These were patients who were well known to the treatment team on the patient care unit. But, we were missing that piece of vital information and a process for addressing it. Once we did that, patients stayed healthier.

4. How about the difference between home care and transitional care?

Again, the emphasis is on empowering the patient for self-management, not on providing care. This was the most difficult thing for the nurses who assumed the transitional care role. Nurses are used to doing things for people; they want to help. It is a shift in paradigm to help by not doing something. It took a lot of practice to "sit on our hands" (as Dr. Coleman's trainers emphasize) and ask patients to show us how they would do something rather than just do it for them.

The other difference is the relationship with the patient begins in the hospital. So, the transition coach or transitional nurse is well acquainted with the hospital course. And our transition staff is part of the hospital team so they have a close working relationship with the physicians, nurses, and ancillary care staff. An unanticipated service our transition staff was able to offer is that of liaison between the home care nurse and the hospital. The homecare nurse often had questions about the hospitalization or why certain things were ordered upon discharge, and our transition staff was able to clear up the confusion. Finally, any patient who met our inclusion criteria could receive coaching services, regardless of payment source or insurance coverage. Our inclusion criteria was very broad. We bent over backward to serve any patient who was receptive.

A Conversation with the Author (cont.)

5. How did your hospital benefit from your transitional programming?

One of the strongest indicators of dissatisfaction for our patients was the discharge process. This is true for many hospitals. Patient satisfaction with our transition programming is very high. Patients tell us it's like having a "daughter who is a nurse." You know, patients feel like there is someone they can trust who is looking out for them and who can explain things they might not understand. Most of our patients in this program ask for "their nurse" whenever they come back to our hospital, even if it is just for something routine like a mammogram. Our transition staff gives the patients in their caseloads a cell number where they can be reached at any time. I can say absolutely that they are never called in the middle of the night for an unimportant issue.

We have also positioned our hospital very well for changes in the payment structure that will penalize high readmission rates and institute the concept of bundling.

6. How did you ensure successful implementation of your transitions programming?

We established our goals and expected outcomes right away and monitored our progress very closely. We talked several times a week about both process and patient issues. We learned from every patient and every encounter and paid attention to the learning process. Once we had data from which we could draw conclusions, we analyzed it very carefully so we could keep doing the things that made us successful and stop doing the things that weren't getting us anywhere.

We also invested in the training provided by Dr. Coleman and Dr. Naylor. Both programs were extremely valuable in getting us off on the right foot and helping us with our struggles along the way. And, last but not least, we shared our success internally and externally. We lasted through some difficult financial times at our hospital because we were widely recognized as contributing something very important to our patients.

To Teach, Learn to Listen

Adults learn more easily when we engage them and build upon previously acquired knowledge. The following guidance is provided as a tool to aid you in the process.

Ask and Listen

• What activities have you stopped doing because of your health? What would you like to be able to do again?

• If you learn more about how a history of stroke (insert applicable disease here) affects your health, do you think you can manage it better?

• Let's begin with what you already know. How do you generally manage your health issues?

Discuss

Now that you have some background information and the patient's attention, it is the right time to begin to offer information. First, present information that is timely and relevant to what they will need to do right away.

Ask and Listen

• Would you agree that, by doing the things we have discussed, you could improve your health?

• How do you think you can incorporate the information I have provided into your daily life?

By following this format, you have:

• Attracted the ATTENTION of the patient.

• Gathered information about what the patient NEEDS.

• Provided FACTS the patient needs to know.

• Gained AGREEMENT that this information presented is important and will help the patient achieve his or her personal goals.

• Encouraged the patient to tell you in his OWN WORDS how he understands and will use the information you have provided.

• Facilitated the development of a PLAN for incorporating health management into the patient's life.

Get Involved! Learn From Colleagues

If you are interested in improving transitions and reducing readmissions, there are some opportunities to learn from other healthcare professionals who are implementing improvements.

Project BOOST (Better Outcomes for Older Adults through Safe Transitions)

This collaborative, coordinated by the Society for Hospital Medicine, began in March 2009. The overall goal was to improve transitions from hospital to home for older adults.

Specific aims included:

- Reduce 30-day readmission rates for general medicine patients (with particular focus on older adults).

- Improve facility patient satisfaction scores.

- Improve the institution's HCAHPS scores related to discharge.

- Improve flow of information between hospital and outpatient physicians.

- Ensure high-risk patients are identified and specific interventions are offered to mitigate their risk.

- Improve patient and family education practices to encourage use of the teach back process around risk-specific issues.

The collaborative process will endeavor to create a national consensus for best practices in transitions from hospital to home, create resources for best practice and provide expert advice in the forms of training sessions and mentoring.

The resources include:

- A clinical toolkit that includes risk stratification and allied plan, a universal set of expectations for all patients being discharged from hospital to home, and a listing of items patients need to be prepared for upon discharge

- A transition record for patients that includes a listing of potential issues and how to resolve them, important contact information, questions for the doctor, and a record of appointments

- An explanation of the teach back process

Get Involved! Learn From Colleagues (cont.)

- Instructions for each intervention applicable to the patient based on the risk identification.

- A format for written discharge instructions

All of the tools, the names of participating hospitals and case studies from participating hospitals are available online at *www.hospitalmedicine.org/ResourceRoomRedesign/RR_CareTransitions/CT_Home.cfm.*

H2H – Hospital to Home

This collaborative is sponsored by the American College of Cardiology and the Institute for Healthcare Improvement. Their broad goal is to create a coordinated team approach across different levels of care for cardiology patients to ensure safe, reliable, health-enhancing transitions. Their specific aim is to reduce the 30-day all-cause readmission rates among patients discharged with heart failure or AMI by 20 percent by December 2012. Although the collaborative has already begun, it is possible to continue to enroll to take advantage of webinars, the listserv and tools provided through this program. Partici-pants are expected to report progress periodically by responding to surveys sent to collaborative members. To learn more and enroll in the collaborative, visit *www.h2hquality.org.*

STAAR – STate Action on Avoidable Rehospitalizations

This is a three-state collaborative facilitated by the Institute for Healthcare Improvement and funded by the Commonwealth Fund. Participants in Michigan, Massachusetts, and Washington are working with payers, patients, families, caregivers, and state and national stakeholders to reduce avoidable hospital readmissions. The goal is to improve transitions between sites of care and reduce fragmentation. The collaborative began on May 1, 2009, so tools and materials being used in the collaborative are now shared on the website. They include:

- A one page summary of the STAAR initiative

- A How-To Guide Summary and Strategies for Getting Started

- STAAR: A State-Based Strategy to Reduce Avoidable Rehospitalizations

- A Survey of the Published Evidence

- A Compendium of Promising Interventions

Get Involved! Learn From Colleagues (cont.)

- STAAR: A Tool for State Policy Makers

- Decreasing Avoidable 30-Day Rehospitalizations: A Mini Course

Visit *www.ihi.org/IHI/Programs/StrategicInitiatives/STateActiononAvoidableRehospitalizationsSTAAR. htm?TabId=0* for more information and to access tools.

Med-IC – Medicare Innovations Collaborative

This collaborative is made up of six healthcare systems dedicated to improving acute and transitional care for complex multimorbid adults. The six healthcare systems are

- Geisinger Health System

- Carolinas Medical Center – Mercy

- Crouse Hospital

- LeHigh Valley Health Network

- Aurora Sinai Medical Center

- University Hospitals Case Medical Center

The healthcare systems are implementing the following programs:

- The Care Transitions Intervention[SM]

- NICHE – Nurses Improving the Care of Healthsystem Elders

- HELP – Hospital Elder Life Program

- ACE – Acute Care for Elders

- Palliative Care

- Hospital at Home

Visit *http://med-ic.org/index.html* to learn more about the sites and the models of care.

Get Involved! Learn From Colleagues (cont.)

Additional Online Resources

Ask Me 3

www.npsf.org/askme3

Ask Me 3 is a patient education program designed to promote communication between healthcare providers by encouraging patients to understand the answers to three questions:

1. What is my main problem?

2. What do I need to do?

3. Why is it important for me to do this?

Care Transitions Intervention℠

www.caretransitions.org

This is the website for the Care Transitions Intervention℠ discussed in Chapter 5: Transitions Programming. It contains tools and resources for implementation.

Centers for Medicare and Medicaid Services Continuity Assessment and Record and Evaluation (CARE)

www.pacdemo.rti.org

The Continuity Assessment Record and Evaluation (CARE) tool, a standardized patient assessment tool, was developed for use at acute hospital discharge and at postacute admission and discharge, as a part of the Post Acute Care Payment Reform Demonstration (PAC-PRD). This site contains the tool, resources, and contact information.

CMS Resources for Caregivers

www.medicare.gov/caregivers

This official Medicare site contains information for caregivers accessing healthcare services.

Get Involved! Learn From Colleagues (cont.)

Evercare

http://evercarehealthplans.com

This is the site for the Evercare Program discussed in Chapter 7: Nursing Home Transitions.

Family Caregiver Alliance

www.caregiver.org/caregiver/jsp/content_node.jsp?nodeid=405

Family Caregiver Alliance (FCA) seeks to improve the quality of life for caregivers through education, services, research, and advocacy. Their website includes publications, teleconferences, toolkits, statistics, and information on public policy initiatives.

Google Health

www.google.com/health

This is a secure, private online health record.

Hartford Institute for Geriatric Nursing

www.consultgerirn.org

This is the evidence-based geriatric clinical nursing website of The Hartford Institute for Geriatric Nursing, at New York University's College of Nursing and NICHE, a program of the Hartford Institute. It contains clinical resources and tools, resources for continuing education and certification, and information on nursing advocacy.

Home Health Quality Improvement

www.homehealthquality.org/hh/default.aspx

This is a grassroots movement designed to unite home health stakeholders and multiple healthcare settings under the shared vision of reducing avoidable hospitalizations and improving medication management. Visitors to the site can join the partnership and find educational resources.

Get Involved! Learn From Colleagues (cont.)

Hospital Compare

www.hospitalcompare.hhs.gov

This tool contains information on hospital quality related to some medical conditions and surgical procedures, as well as results from a survey of patients about the quality of care patients received during a recent hospital stay.

Improving Chronic Care

www.improvingchroniccare.org

Information on the chronic care model and resources related to caring for patients with chronic illness is provided on this site.

INTERACT II (Improve Care and Reduce Acute Care Transfers)

http://interact.geriu.org

Contained in this site is information on implementing INTERACT II, including the toolkit discussed in Chapter 7: Nursing Home Transitions.

Microsoft Health Vault

www.healthvault.com

This is a secure, private online health record.

National Council on Patient Information and Education

www.healthfinder.gov/orgs/HR1913.htm

The National Council on Patient Information and Education (NCPIE) is a nonprofit coalition of over 120 government, consumer, patient advocacy, and public health organizations whose mission it is to stimulate and improve communication of information on the appropriate use of medicines between healthcare professionals and consumers. The site contains information and interactive tools.

Get Involved! Learn From Colleagues (cont.)

National Family Caregivers Association

www.nfcacares.org

This Association educates, supports, empowers and speaks up for the more than 65 million Americans who care for loved ones with a chronic illness or disability or the frailties of old age. The site contains information, resources, and an online support group.

Next Step In Care

www.nextstepincare.org

This site provides information and advice to help family caregivers and healthcare providers plan safe and smooth transitions for patients. Tools for healthcare providers and family caregivers are included.

Patient Activation Measure

www.insigniahealth.com

This is the site for the Patient Activation Measure™ (PAM™) discussed in Chapter 3: Patient Self-Management, which assesses the knowledge, skills, and confidence integral to managing one's own health and healthcare. It contains information on patient activation and self-management.

Peace Health's Shared Care Plan

www.sharedcareplan.org

This is a secure, private online health record.

Physician Consortium for Performance Improvement

www.ama-assn.org/ama/pub/physician-resources/clinical-practice-improvement/clinical-quality/
physician-consortium-performance-improvement.shtml

The American Medical Association (AMA) -convened Physician Consortium for Performance Improvement (PCPI®) is committed to enhancing quality of care and patient safety by taking the lead in the development, testing, and maintenance of evidence-based clinical performance measures and measurement resources for physicians. Their site contains resources, position papers, and performance measures for 42 clinical topics and conditions.

Get Involved! Learn From Colleagues (cont.)

Project RED

www.bu.edu/fammed/projectred

This is the site for Project RED, discussed in Chapter 4: Reengineering the Hospital Discharge.

Quality Improvement Organizations

www.ipro.org/index/care-links

This is the site for one of the CMS quality improvement organizations charged with improving care transitions in its community. Activities of the collaborative, along with an extensive list of resources are provided.

Questions Are the Answer

www.ahrq.gov/questionsaretheanswer

This site, sponsored by the Agency for Healthcare Research and Quality, encourages patients to become more active participants in their healthcare. Information on talking with clinicians, understanding medical tests and planning for surgery are provided. An online question builder is provided.

Telehealth – Veterans Affairs

www.carecoordination.va.gov/telehealth

This site provides an overview of Telehealth for patients.

The Medicare Payment Advisory Committee

www.medpac.gov

MedPac advises Congress on Medicare issues. This site includes information on upcoming meetings and reports.

Get Involved! Learn From Colleagues (cont.)

The National Transitions of Care Coalition

www.ntocc.org

The National Transitions of Care Coalition (NTOCC) brings together thought leaders, patient advocates, and healthcare providers from various care settings dedicated to improving the quality of care coordination and communication during patient transfer from one level of care to another. Their website contains information for consumers, healthcare providers, and policymakers.

The Newest Vital Sign

www.pfizerhealthliteracy.com/physicians-providers/newest-vital-sign.html

This is the site for the assessment of health literacy discussed in Chapter 3: Patient Self-Management.

Transitional Care

www.transitionalcare.info/index.html

This is the site for the Transitional Care Model discussed in Chapter 5: Transitions Programming.

A Personal Message From the Author

So, you have decided you'd like to implement a program to reduce readmissions. How do you convince your CEO? Mine told me I could sell ice to Eskimos so I thought I'd pass along a few tips for selling your idea.

1. Get Her Attention

Once you have figured out why your organization can't live another day without a program, gather data and present it as succinctly as possible. Say something provocative like, "Did you know that 50% of patients do not take their medications correctly? And, that often causes a readmission?" Develop an elevator speech – something you can say to a key decision maker as quickly as it takes to ride in an elevator.

2. Describe the Need

Now that you have the attention of the CEO, describe your organization's need for a program in a factual and data-based way. There are several good studies supporting the need for and outcomes of these programs. Many of them are cited in this book. Refer to them in this section of your presentation.

3. Review the Facts

Tell your CEO what you'd like to do. Let her know that you have thought through how the program would be implemented in your organization.

4. Get Agreement

Check to see whether your CEO agrees that there is a need and this program will fulfill that need. Encourage her to voice any concerns and ask questions. This will give you the opportunity to put any lingering doubts she has to rest.

5. Close

This is the most overlooked part of the sales pitch, probably because it is hard to do. But, make sure you close the sale. Ask her for the organizational support to implement your program. If she is reluctant to fully implement the program, she might be more receptive to a pilot. You will be able to prove your worth so there is no shame is beginning this way.

I know you can do it. Get out there and get started!

Continuing Education Instructional Guide

Reducing Readmissions: A Blueprint for Improving Care Transitions

Target Audience

Directors of case management

Hospital case managers

Nurses

Statement of Need

As healthcare reforms are implemented, it will be in the best interest of providers to prevent hospital readmissions and enhance transitional care through collaboration and patient self-management. This book provides a practical overview of several innovative and effective programs to reduce readmissions and suggestions for implementing these programs based on sound leadership practices.

Educational Objectives

Upon completion of this activity, participants should be able to:

1. Identify the leading components of quality transitional care.

2. Explain the role healthcare technology should play in enhancing the transition process.

3. Identify and discuss the issues associated with patient noncompliance.

4. Describe patient-centered care in chronic disease.

5. Define patient self-management.

6. Describe the characteristics of an adult learning model.

7. Identify the levels of patient activation and the appropriate teaching methods associated with each.

8. Define literacy and health literacy and discuss the issues associated with low levels of both in the chronically ill adult population.

9. Identify the most frequent adverse events that occur after a hospitalization and their causes.

10. Describe the RED process, including its 11 components.

11. Define the roles of discharge advocate and embodied conversational advocate.

12. Describe two care transitions programs, including the role of the transition coach and transitional care nurse.

13. Identify expected outcomes from transitional programming.

14. Summarize practical considerations for implementing a transitions program.

15. Discuss the value of caregiving to society and the personal cost to the caregiver.

16. Evaluate caregiver assessments and incorporate one into your practice.

17. Describe the elements of an educational process for caregivers.

18. Identify the causes of acute care transfers from nursing homes and the potential problems for residents.

19. Discuss three programs for addressing acute care transfers from nursing homes and their emerging evidence base.

20. Evaluate the potential for implementation of the INTERACT II toolkit.

21. Define cultural and linguistic competence and outline its impact on healthcare organizations.

22. Identify mandated and suggested standards for providing culturally competent care.

23. Analyze methods for implementing various programs to reduce readmissions.

24. Describe a process for introducing innovation into an organization.

Faculty

Lead author:

Christina Pavetto Bond, MS, FACHE—Director, Aging and Complex Care

Crouse Hospital, Syracuse, NY

Contributing author:

Eric Coleman, MD, MPH

Division of Healthcare Policy and Research at University of Colorado, Denver

Nursing Contact Hours

HCPro, Inc., is accredited as a provider of continuing nursing education by the American Nurses Credentialing Center's Commission on Accreditation.

This educational activity for 3.5 nursing contact hours is provided by HCPro, Inc.

Commission for Case Manager Certification (CCMC)

This program is approved by the Commission for Case Manager Certification for 4 Continuing Education Units.

Disclosure Statements

HCPro, Inc., has confirmed that none of the faculty, planners, or contributors have any relevant financial relationships to disclose related to the content of this educational activity.

Disclosure of Unlabeled Use

This educational activity may contain discussion of published and/or investigational uses of agents that are not indicated by the FDA. HCPro, Inc., does not recommend the use of any agent outside of the labeled indications. The opinions expressed in the educational activity are those of the faculty and do not necessarily represent the views of HCPro, Inc. Please refer to the official prescribing information for each product for discussion of approved indications, contraindications, and warnings.

Instructions

In order to be eligible to receive your nursing contact hours or case manager continuing education credits for this activity, you are required to do the following:

1. Read the book, *Reducing Readmissions: A Blueprint for Improving Care Transitions*

2. Complete the exam and receive a passing score of 80%.

3. Complete the evaluation.

4. Provide your contact information on the exam and evaluation.

5. Submit exam and evaluation to HCPro, Inc.

Please provide all of the information requested above and mail or fax your completed exam, program evaluation, and contact information to:

HCPro, Inc.

Attention: Continuing Education Manager

P.O. Box 1168

Marblehead, MA 01945

Fax: 781/639-2982

NOTE:

This book and associated exam are intended for individual use only. If you would like to provide this continuing education exam to other members of your nursing or physician staff, please contact our customer service department at 877/727-1728 to place your order. The exam fee schedule is as follows:

Exam quantity	Fee
1	$0
2–25	$15 per person
26–50	$12 per person
51–100	$8 per person
101+	$5 per person

Continuing Education Exam

Name: _____

Title: _____

Facility name: _____

Address: _____

Address: _____

City: _____ State: _____ ZIP: _____

Phone number: _____ Fax number: _____

E-mail: _____

Date completed: _____

1. **How many Medicare beneficiaries are readmitted to the hospital within 30 days?**

   a. 1 in 5

   b. 1 in 10

   c. 1 in 15

   d. 1 in 20

2. **Telehealth involves the use of technology to remotely engage and evaluate patients, particularly those who:**

   a. Live in urban areas

   b. Live in rural or frontier settings

   c. Have learning disabilities

   d. Have multiple illnesses

3. **The World Health Organization (WHO) estimates that as many as _____% of patients fail to take medications correctly:**

    a. 30

    b. 40

    c. 50

    d. 80

4. **The Chronic Care Model identifies the essential elements of a healthcare system that:**

    a. Encourages high-quality chronic disease care

    b. Encourages high-quality physician care

    c. Improves the patient's success with treatment

    d. Improves the hospital's revenue

5. **Which of the following does The Disease Management Association of America emphasize as central to chronic disease intervention?**

    a. Availability of clinical staff

    b. Efficient scheduling of patient appointments

    c. More home visits and medication counseling

    d. Patient self-management

6. **Pedagogical methods, for the most part, are:**

    a. Patient-directed

    b. Teacher-directed

    c. Physician-directed

    d. Child-directed

7. **"Patient activation" is defined as patients' levels of knowledge, skill, and confidence regarding their ability to:**

    a. Take care of themselves without any further assistance

    b. Become more physically active

    c. Communicate effectively with their physicians

    d. Manage their own health and healthcare

8. **Inadequate health literacy has been associated with:**

    a. Difficulty in effective communication

    b. Poor health outcomes

    c. Patient apathy

    d. An inability to read

9. **Which of the following have studies shown to be the cause of poorly conducted acute long-term care transitions?**

    a. Poor communication

    b. High staff turnover

    c. Patients' refusal to comply

    d. Lack of electronic personal health records

10. **Project RED's embodied conversational agent can be used to educate all patients, but is particularly useful for individuals with:**

    a. Learning disabilities

    b. Physical limitations

    c. Low health literacy

    d. Chronic disease

11. **A fundamental role of the discharge advocate is to:**

    a. Educate patients throughout their stay regarding their diagnosis

    b. Educate patients after their stay regarding their diagnosis

    c. Teach patients how to avoid taking medication

    d. Provide counseling to the patients' family members

12. **Transition coaches:**

    a. Provide skilled care to the patient

    b. Provide financial guidance to the patient

    c. Provide transition information and guidance to the patient

    d. None of the above

13. **In Mary Naylor's Transitional Care model, a home visit typically occurs:**

    a. Within 24 to 48 hours of discharge

    b. Within 48 to 72 hours of discharge

    c. One week after discharge

    d. Three weeks after discharge

14. **The transitional care nurse acts as the primary coordinator of care:**

    a. During the entire episode of care, including the hospital stay

    b. During the hospital stay and up to one month following discharge

    c. Only during the hospital stay

    d. Only after discharge

15. **Which of the following outcomes should be expected from transitional programming?**

    a. Decline in medication discrepancies

    b. Increased patient satisfaction

    c. Reduction in hospital readmissions

    d. All of the above

16. **People who have caregivers tend to have:**

    a. Fewer medications

    b. Shorter hospital stays

    c. Less serious illness

    d. Greater health literacy

17. **Which statement about educating caregivers is inaccurate?**

    a. When possible, teach the caregiver at the bedside using equipment and supplies he will use at home.

    b. Be sure the caregiver knows your intent is to help him with information that will be useful.

    c. Emphasize the things the caregiver will need to know for the next two years of caregiving.

    d. Ask the caregiver to repeat what he understands about what you have told him.

18. **In improving nursing home-emergency department transitions, what is the primary issue to address?**

    a. Patients who do not understand their self-care and their medications

    b. Lack of collaboration and miscommunication between the clinical teams at each facility

    c. Staff members who work too slowly

    d. None of the above

19. **Use of the INTERACT II tools begins when:**

    a. The resident is admitted

    b. The resident is discharged

    c. The staff notices a change in the resident's status

    d. The resident's condition beings to improve

20. **The SBAR tool helps to improve communication between the treatment team members by providing guidelines that ensure all members:**

    a. Use the same approach with each patient

    b. Use consistent language

    c. Spend equal amounts of time with each patient

    d. None of the above

21. **Among adults age 50 and older, which of the following racial groups is most likely to have at least one of the most common chronic conditions?**

    a. White

    b. Latino

    c. Asian

    d. There is no distinction among races in chronic illness.

22. **How many standards have the U.S. Department of Health and Human Services set forth for culturally and linguistically appropriate services?**

    a. 10

    b. 14

    c. 22

    d. 25

23. **Most experts recommend beginning the process of implementing a new practice by:**

    a. Analyzing the environment in which the new process will function

    b. Assessing the organization's finances and budget

    c. Determining the level of employee commitment to implement a new process

    d. Selecting team members to start the process

24. **Which of the following statements is inaccurate regarding readmission program implementation?**

    a. In general, it is difficult to implement major change initiatives without investing in its infrastructure.

    b. Leaders of the change should not open themselves up to questions and concerns from staff.

    c. The process of innovation and leadership team should be supported by a sponsor.

    d. Structure, process, and outcome are important quality measurement considerations.

Continuing Education Exam Answer Key

Name: _____ License #: _____

Facility: _____ Title: _____

Address: _____

City: _____ State: _____ Zip: _____

Phone: _____ E-mail: _____

(Certificates are emailed to learners unless otherwise stated here)

Please record the letter of the correct answer to the corresponding exam question below:					
1.	5.	9.	13.	17.	21.
2.	6.	10.	14.	18.	22.
3.	7.	11.	15.	19.	23.
4.	8.	12.	16.	20.	24.

Continuing Education Evaluation

1 = Strongly Agree	**2** = Agree	**3** = Disagree	**4** = Strongly Disagree

(Please rate the responses below according to the scale above to rate the quality of this educational activity)

1. **Please indicate how well you feel this activity met the learning objectives listed:** 1 2 3 4

2. **Objectives were related to the overall purpose/goal of the activity:** 1 2 3 4

3. **This activity was related to my continuing education needs:** 1 2 3 4

4. **The exam for the activity was an accurate test of the knowledge gained:** 1 2 3 4

5.   The activity avoided commercial bias or influence: 1   2   3   4

6.   This activity met my expectations: 1   2   3   4

7.   The format was an appropriate method for delivery of the
     content for this activity: 1   2   3   4

8.   Will this activity enhance your professional practice?   Yes   No

9.   How much time did it take for you to complete this activity?   _____

10. Do you have any additional comments on this activity?

     _____

     _____

     _____

     _____

     _____

Return completed form to:
HCPro, Inc. · Attention: Continuing Education Manager · P.O. Box 1168, Marblehead, MA 01945 ·
Telephone: 877/727-1728 · Fax: 781/639-2982

FREE HEALTHCARE COMPLIANCE AND MANAGEMENT RESOURCES!

Need to control expenses yet stay current with critical issues?

Get timely help with FREE e-mail newsletters from HCPro, Inc., the leader in healthcare compliance education. Offering numerous free electronic publications covering a wide variety of essential topics, you'll find just the right e-newsletter to help you stay current, informed, and effective. All you have to do is sign up!

With your FREE subscriptions, you'll also receive the following:

- Timely information, to be read when convenient with your schedule

- Expert analysis you can count on

- Focused and relevant commentary

- Tips to make your daily tasks easier

And here's the best part: There's no further obligation—just a complimentary resource to help you get through your daily challenges.

It's easy. Visit *www.hcmarketplace.com/free/e-newsletters* to register for as many free e-newsletters as you'd like, and let us do the rest.

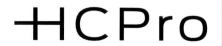

HCPro | Insight for healthcare compliance and management